Chairman and editor: Wolfgang Schultze, Bad Saarow

High-Dose Therapy and Transplantation of Haematopoietic Stem Cells (2001)

Proceedings of the 5th International Stem Cell Workshop:

High-Dose Therapy and Transplantation of Haematopoietic Stem Cells (2001)

(Bad Saarow/Berlin, Germany, April 26-28, 2001)

Chairman and editor: Wolfgang Schultze, Bad Saarow

With 39 Figures and 40 Tables

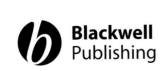

Blackwell
Publishing

1st English-language edition:
© 2002 by Blackwell Verlag Berlin · Vienna
A Blackwell Publishing Company

Editorial Offices:
Blackwell Publishing Ltd
Osney Mead, Oxford, OX2 0EL, UK
108 Cowley Road, Oxford, OX4 1JF, UK

Blackwell Publishing, Inc.
350 Main Street, Malden,
MA 02148-5018, USA

Blackwell Publishing Asia Pty Ltd
550 Swanston Street, Carlton
Victoria 3053, Australia

Blackwell Verlag GmbH
Kurfürstendamm 57, 10707 Berlin, Germany
Firmiangasse 7, 1130 Wien, Austria

Editor's address:
Dozent Dr. med. habil. W. Schultze
HUMAINE Klinikum
Klinik für Innere Medizin
15526 Bad Saarow
Germany

A catalogue record for this title
is available from the British Library
and the Library of Congress

ISBN 1-4051-0019-2

Cover design: Petry & Schwamb,
Emmendingen (using Fig. 6.4-2)
Production and set by: Schröders Agentur
Printed and bound by: Druckhaus Köthen

The right of the Authors to be identified as
the Authors of this work has been asserted
in accordance with the German Copyright
Law of September 9, 1965, in its version of
June, 1985.

For further information on Blackwell Science,
visit our website: www.blackwell-science.com

Preface

The question, still prevailing at the 5th International Stem Cell Workshop, centred, once again, on the future role attributed to (i) aggressive high-dose anti-cancer therapy and (ii) autologous or allogeneic stem cell transplantation.

Among the experts in the field, there was almost unanimous agreement as to the necessity of aggressive strategies in the therapy of certain malignant diseases. There is, nevertheless, a very strong quest for less aggressive forms of treatment with abating side effects. This was highlighted by novel strategies for further achievements in, for example, non-myeloablative therapy of haematologic malignancies or solid tumours with subsequent allogeneic stem cell grafts, or adoptive immunotherapy, or gene therapy.

Autologous stem cell transplantation is, no doubt, receding; the expectations were too high, and the unfortunate manoeuvres to which high-dose therapy of breast cancer had been exposed were eventually detrimental to further attempts with other solid tumours. Conversely, there was a sense of trust with respect to advances in allogeneic stem cell transplantation for solid tumours with poor prognosis.

Multiple myeloma was the object of promising approaches, using allogeneic as well as autologous stem cell application with reduced myeloablation.

At present, progress in the field is highlighted by novel treatment strategies which exploit immunological techniques and genetic engineering. Future prospects and tools will include the introduction of new pharmaceuticals, mesenchymal stem cells, and biological factors in order to improve cancer therapy. For the time being, the 5th Workshop offered an additional opportunity to become acquainted with the present state of the art of stem cell transplantation.

The editor wishes to thank the authors for their contributions, and M. Hess for his kind assistance.

Bad Saarow, Spring 2002   Wolfgang Schultze

Table of Contents

Part Three Management of Graft-versus-Host Disease

Part Four   Miscellaneous / Short Communications*

Contributors

Abken, H.
Klinik I für Innere Medizin
Labor für Tumorgenetik
University of Cologne
50924 Cologne
Germany

Baum, C.
Dept. of Tumour Virology
Heinrich Pette Institute
20251 Hamburg
and
Dept. of Haematology and Oncology
Hanover Medical School
30625 Hanover
Germany

Blume, K.
Stanford University
Stanford, CA
U.S.A.

Buxhofer, V.
2nd Dept. of Medicine
Ludwig Boltzmann Institute for
Stem Cell Transplantation
Donauspital/SMZO
1220 Vienna
Austria

Casper, J.
Dept. of Haematology and Oncology
University of Rostock
18057 Rostock
Germany

Czaika, V.A.
HUMAINE Klinikum
Klinik für Innere Medizin
15526 Bad Saarow
Germany

Derigs, G.
University Hospital
Johannes Gutenberg University
55116 Mainz
Germany

Dreger, P.
2nd Dept. of Medicine
University of Kiel
24116 Kiel
Germany

Düllmann, J.
Dept. of Neuroanatomy
Eppendorf University Hospital
University of Hamburg
20251 Hamburg
Germany

Eckert, H.-G.
European Institute for Research and
Development of Transplantation
Strategies (EUFETS GmbH)
55743 Idar-Oberstein
and
Dept. of Haematology and Oncology
Hanover Medical School
30625 Hanover
Germany

Ehninger, G.
Medizinische Klinik und Poliklinik I
Univ.-Klinikum Carl Gustav Carus
01307 Dresden
Germany

Einsele, H.
Department of Medicine II
University of Tübingen
72076 Tübingen
Germany

Fauser, A.A.
Dept. of Haematology/Oncology and
Bone Marrow Transplantation
55743 Idar-Oberstein
Germany

Fehse, B.
Dept. of Oncology, Haematology and
Bone Marrow Transplantation
Eppendorf University Hospital
University of Hamburg
20251 Hamburg
Germany

Finke, J.
Abt. Hämatologie & Onkologie
Medizinische Universitätsklinik
Freiburg
79106 Freiburg
Germany

Freund, M.
Dept. of Haematology and Oncology
University of Rostock
18057 Rostock
Germany

Gösta Gahrton
Dept. of Medicine and Haematology
Huddinge University Hospital
Stockholm
Sweden

Görner, M.
Dept. of Haematology/Oncology/
Rheumatology
University of Heidelberg
69115 Heidelberg
Germany

Goldschmidt, H.
Department of Internal Medicine V
University of Heidelberg
Hospitalstr. 3
69115 Heidelberg
Germany

Gutensohn, K.
Blood Transfusion Service
Eppendorf University Hospital
20246 Hamburg
Germany

Haas, R.
Dept. of Haematology, Oncology and
Clinical Immunology
Heinrich Heine University
40225 Düsseldorf
Germany

Hegenbart, U.
University of Leipzig
04103 Leipzig
Germany

Held, T. K.
Abt. für Innere Medizin und Poliklinik
Schwerpunkt Hämatologie/Onkologie
Univ.-Klinikum Charité, Campus
Virchow
13353 Berlin
Germany

Hinke, A.
WISP Research Institute
40764 Langenfeld
Germany

Hinterberger, W.
2nd Dept. of Medicine
Ludwig Boltzmann Institute for
Stem Cell Transplantation
Donauspital/SMZO
1220 Vienna
Austria

Ho, A. D.
Dept. of Haematology/Oncology/
Rheumatology
University of Heidelberg
69115 Heidelberg
Germany

Hombach, A.
Klinik I für Innere Medizin
Labor für Tumorgenetik
University of Cologne
50924 Cologne
Germany

Jänicke, F.
Dept. of Gynaecology and Obstetrics
Eppendorf University Hospital
20246 Hamburg
Germany

Jung, R.
Dept. of Clinical Chemistry
Eppendorf University Hospital
20246 Hamburg
Germany

Knauf, W. U.
Bone Marrow Transplantation Unit
Dept. of Medicine III (Haematology,
Oncology and Transfusion Medicine)
Universitätsklinikum Benjamin
Franklin
Freie Universität Berlin
12200 Berlin
Germany

Kobbe, G. P.
Dept. of Haematology, Oncology and
Clinical Immunology
Heinrich Heine University
40225 Düsseldorf
Germany

Koch, St.
HUMAINE Klinikum
Institut für Pathologie
15526 Bad Saarow
Germany

Kolb, H. J.
Haematopoietic Cell Transplantation
José Carreras Transplantation Unit
Klinikum University of Munich-
Grosshadern
81377 Munich
Germany

Kröger, N.
Bone Marrow Transplantation Unit
Dept. of Oncology/Haematology
Eppendorf University Hospital
University of Hamburg
20251 Hamburg
Germany

Kronenwett, R.
Dept. of Haematology, Oncology and
Clinical Immunology
University of Düsseldorf
40225 Düsseldorf
Germany

Krüger, W. H.
Bone Marrow Transplantation Unit
Dept. of Oncology/Haematology
Eppendorf University Hospital
University of Hamburg
20246 Hamburg
Germany
and
Dept. of Haematology and Oncology
Internal Medicine IV
Martin Luther University
Halle-Wittenberg
06108 Halle/Saale
Germany

Krüll, A.
Dept. of Radiotherapy
Eppendorf University Hospital
University of Hamburg
20246 Hamburg
Germany

Kuse, R.
Dept. of Haematology
A. K. St. Georg
20099 Hamburg
Germany

Leiblein, S.
Div. of Haematology/Oncology
University of Leipzig
04103 Leipzig
Germany

Leskovar, P.
Immunol.-Biochem. Res. Laboratory
Dept. of Urology
Medical School, Technical University
Munich
Germany

Li, Z.
Dept. of Tumour Virology
Heinrich Pette Institute
20251 Hamburg

Löliger, C.
Dept. of Transfusion Medicine
Eppendorf University Hospital
University of Hamburg
20246 Hamburg
Germany

McSweeney, P.A.
University of Colorado
Health Sciences Center
Colorado

Martin, S.
Dept. of Haematology, Oncology and
Clinical Immunology
University of Düsseldorf
40225 Düsseldorf
Germany

Moehler, T. M.
Dept. of Haematology/Oncology/
Rheumatology
University of Heidelberg
69115 Heidelberg
Germany

Neubauer, A.
Dept. of Haematology
Klinikum der Philips-Universität
35037 Marburg
Germany

Niederwieser, D.
Div. of Haematology/Oncology
University of Leipzig
04103 Leipzig
Germany

Pape, H.
Dept. of Radiotherapy
Heinrich Heine University
40225 Düsseldorf
Germany

Pönisch, W.
Div. of Haematology/Oncology
University of Leipzig
04103 Leipzig
Germany

Schäfer, P.
Dept. of Transfusion Medicine
Eppendorf University Hospital
University of Hamburg
20246 Hamburg
Germany

Schäfer, U. W.
Bone Marrow Transplantation Unit
University Hospital
45122 Essen
Germany

Schäfer-Eckart, K.
Bone Marrow Transplantation Unit
Städtisches Klinikum
90400 Nürnberg
Germany

Schetelig, J.
Abt. für Innere Medizin and Poliklinik
Schwerpunkt Hämatologie/Onkologie
Univ.-Klinikum Charité, Campus
Virchow
13353 Berlin
Germany

Schmalreck, A. F.
Mikrobiological Service Munich
80993 Munich
Germany

Schmidmaier, R.
Immunol.-Biochem. Res. Laboratory
Dept. of Urology
Medical School
Technical University
Munich
Germany

Schmitz, F.
Dept. of Haematology and Oncology
Johannes Gutenberg University
55116 Mainz
Germany

Schultze, W.
HUMAINE Klinikum
Klinik für Innere Medizin
15526 Bad Saarow
Germany

Schwerdtfeger, R.
Bone Marrow Transplantation Unit
Deutsche Klinik für Diagnostik
65000 Wiesbaden
Germany

Siegert, W.
Abt. für Innere Medizin and Poliklinik
Schwerpunkt Hämatologie/Onkologie
Univ.-Klinikum Charité, Campus
Virchow
13353 Berlin
Germany

Storb, R.
Fred Hutchinson Cancer Research
Center
Seattle, WA 98109-1024
and
University of Washington
Seattle, WA
U.S.A.

Theobald, M.
Dept. of Haematology and Oncology
Johannes Gutenberg University
55116 Mainz
Germany

Thiel, E.
Bone Marrow Transplantation Unit
Dept. of Medicine III (Haematology,
Oncology and Transfusion Medicine)
Universitätsklinikum Benjamin
Franklin
Freie Universität Berlin
12200 Berlin
Germany

Voss, R. H.
Dept. of Haematology and Oncology
Johannes Gutenberg University
55116 Mainz
Germany

Wandt, H.
Bone Marrow Transplantation Unit
Städtisches Klinikum
90400 Nürnberg
Germany

Wegener, H.
Dept. of Forensic Medicine
University of Rostock
18055 Rostock
Germany

Zabelina, T.
Bone Marrow Transplantation Unit
Dept. of Oncology/Haematology
Eppendorf University Hospital
University of Hamburg
20251 Hamburg
Germany

Zander, A. R.
Dept. of Oncology, Haematology and
Bone Marrow Transplantation
Eppendorf University Hospital
University of Hamburg
20251 Hamburg
Germany

Part One
Non-Myeloablative Stem Cell Transplantation

1.1 Haematopoietic Cell Transplantation from Siblings in Older Patients with Haematologic Malignancies: Replacing High-Dose Cytotoxic Therapy with Graft-versus-Tumour Effects

Storb[1,2]*, R., B. M. Sandmaier[1,2], S. Forman[4], M. Maris[1,2], L. Feinstein[1,2], T. Chauncey[1,2,3], D. G. Maloney[1,2], P. A. McSweeney[5], K. G. Blume[6], J. Shizuru[6], U. Hegenbart[7], M.-T. Little[1], D. Niederwieser[7]

[1] Fred Hutchinson Cancer Research Center, [2] University of Washington School of Medicine, [3] Veterans Administration Medical Center, Seattle, WA; [4] City of Hope National Medical Center, [5] University of Colorado Health Sciences Center, [6] Stanford University School of Medicine, Stanford, CA; [7] University of Leipzig, Leipzig, Germany.

*To whom correspondence should be addressed (rstorb@fhcrc.org.)

Supported in part by grants HL36444, HL03701, CA18221, CA15704, CA78902, CA49605 and DK42716 from the National Institutes of Health, DHHS, Bethesda, MD, USA. Support was also provided by the Gabriella Rich Leukemia Foundation. R.S. also received support from the Laura Landro Salomon Endowment Fund, and through a prize awarded by the Josef Steiner Krebsstiftung, Bern, Switzerland.

The finding by JACOBSON *et al.* [4] in 1949, that mice could be protected from the marrow lethal effects of ionizing total body irradiation (TBI) by shielding their spleens with lead marked the start of the modern era of haematopoietic stem cell transplantation (HSCT). Subsequent animal experiments showed in 1956 that the radioprotection was effected by transplantable HSC [3,7,10]. Further studies in large random-bred animal species resulted in the development of HSCT schemas for human patients with marrow-based diseases, such as leukaemias [17]. The schemas involved treatment with very high doses of systemic chemoradiation to eradicate the patients' underlying diseases, followed by HSCT "rescue".

The therapy's intensity would be limited only by serious toxicities to non-marrow organs, such as gut, lung, kidney, heart, and liver.

Most current HSCT approaches are based on the original treatment schemas. However, at least two findings have raised questions whether the treatment schemas are universally valid. One is that many haematological malignancies cannot be wiped out by high-dose chemoradiation, even though therapy has been intensified to levels at which serious organ toxicities are encountered [2,17]. The other is that many of the observed cures seem to be due to immunological graft-versus-tumour reactions [1,8,18,19]. Consequently, donor lymphocyte infusions are now frequently used to reinduce remissions in patients who relapsed after conventional HSCT [5]. The two findings, combined with the observation that regimen-related toxicities have limited conventional HSCT to younger patients with good organ function, and better ways to control both host and donor immune functions, have led to a reassessment of how allogeneic HSCT might be done in the future. For example, instead of trying to eradicate tumours through intensive and toxic chemoradiation, the HSCT donor's immune cells might be used for that purpose, invoking graft-versus-tumour effects. Removing the high-dose chemoradiation from transplant regimens would allow extending HSCT to include those patients who are too old or medically infirm to qualify for conventional allotransplants.

The non-myeloablative HSCT approach used in Seattle, Palo Alto, Duarte, Denver, and Leipzig was based on two experimental observations showing that both host-versus-graft (HvG) and graft-versus-host (GvH) reactions are effected by T-lymphocytes in major histocompatibility complex (MHC) identical HSCT. This has allowed identifying post-transplant immunosuppression which not only controls GvHD but also residual HvG reactions, and, thus, eliminates the need for intensive and potentially organ-toxic pretransplant chemoradiation. Studies in a preclinical canine model explored substituting non-myelotoxic post-transplant immunosuppression for cytotoxic pre-transplant TBI in a stepwise fashion [12,20]. The new transplant schema that evolved from these studies combines some host immunosuppression before and an extended course of immunosuppression after HSCT, which reduces the risk of serious GvHD and eliminates residual HvG responses. Once post-transplant immunosuppression is discontinued, mutual graft-host tolerance may develop, manifesting itself as either stable mixed donor/host or all donor haematopoietic chimerism.

A well-tolerated and effective HSCT regimen in dogs combines a low and non-myeloablative dose of 200 cGy TBI (given at the very low rate of 7 cGy/min) before, with the *de novo* purine synthesis inhibitor mycophenolate mofetil (MMF) and the T-cell activation blocker, cyclosporine (CSP), for 4 and 5 weeks, respectively, after DLA-identical HSCT [12]. Successful allografts are also seen when dogs are given pre-transplant irradiation targeted to cervical, thoracic, and upper abdominal lymph nodes instead of TBI [13]. In these dogs, donor cells establish themselves as early as 6 weeks after HSCT even in lead-shielded, non-irradiated marrow and lymph node sites. This finding challenges the long-held notion that "creation of marrow space" by cytotoxic agents is needed to establish stable allografts, and indicates that the grafts can create their own space through subclinical GvH reactions. It also raises the hope that future regimens may include non-toxic T-cell immunosuppression instead of low-dose pre-transplant TBI. A first step in this direction has been taken in studies in which blockage of T-cell co-stimulation through CTLA4Ig, along with concurrent stimulation of the T-cell receptor with HSC donor antigen, resulted in lowering of the pre-transplant TBI dose needed for stable allografts from 200 cGy to 100 cGy [14].

A new conceptual schema for allogeneic HSCT in patients with malignant haematological diseases was developed on the basis of the preclinical canine studies [15,16]. Initial mixed chimerism was expected to either spontaneously convert to all-donor chimerism during episodes of acute GvHD or after an infusion of donor lymphocytes. The concept has been successfully applied to treat patients with acute and chronic leukaemias, myelodysplasia, Hodgkin's and non-Hodgkin's lymphoma, and multiple myeloma who were ineligible for conventional transplants because of age or medical infirmity [6]. The regimen included a single fraction of pre-transplant TBI, 200 cGy, given at 7 cGy/min, CSP given at 6.25 mg/kg/b.i.d. p.o. on days −3 to 35, with subsequent taper through day 56, and MMF at 15 mg/kg/b.i.d. p.o. beginning in the afternoon of day 0 through day 27. G-CSF mobilized unmodified peripheral blood stem cells (PBSC) were transplanted on day 0. Eighty-eight patients (median age 44 years, range 21–71 years) received PBSC transplants from HLA-matched sibling donors [6,11]. Non-fatal graft rejection occurred among 11 of the first 60 (18%) patients. With the addition of three doses of fludarabine before TBI, all 28 subsequent patients had stable engraftment. Fatal progression of the underlying disease occurred among 18 (20%) patients. Non-relapse mortality was seen in 10 (11%) patients. Grade II–IV acute GvHD occurred among 47%, with 4% of the patients developing grade IV acute GvHD. Chronic GvHD was seen in 46 of 71 (65%) evaluable patients. With a median follow-up of 244 (range 100–842) days, 60 patients (68%) were alive with 37 patients (42%) in complete remission of their underlying diseases.

Under a protocol which extended the postgrafting immunosuppression with MMF and CSP to 96 and 180 days, respectively, 36 patients with a median age of 48 (range 6–65) years received HLA-matched unrelated donor HSCT, after conditioning with fludarabine and 2 Gy TBI [9]. The incidence of rejection was 11%. Acute GvHD occurred in 20 (56%) patients, in all of whom it was of grade II severity. Non-relapse mortality was seen in three (8%) patients, and four (11%) died of relapse. With a median follow-up of 167 (range 18–427) days, 27 (75%) patients were alive, with 20 (56%) patients in complete remission.

References

1. BARNES, D.W.H., LOUTIT, J.F.: Treatment of murine leukaemia with x-rays and homologous bone marrow: II, Br J Hematol 3 (1957) 241.
2. BURCHENAL, J.H., et al.: Effect of total body irradiation on the transplantability of mouse leukemias, Cancer Res 20 (1960) 425.
3. FORD, C.E., et al.: Cytological identification of radiation-chimaeras, Nature 177 (1956) 452.
4. JACOBSON, L.O., et al.: Effect of spleen protection on mortality following x-irradiation, J Lab Clin Med 34 (1949) 1538.
5. KOLB, H.J., et al.: Graft-versus-leukemia effect of donor lymphocyte transfusions in marrow grafted patients. European Group for Blood and Marrow Transplantation Working Party Chronic Leukemia, Blood 86 (1995) 2041.
6. MCSWEENEY, P.A., et al.: Hematopoietic cell transplantation in older patients with hematologic malignancies: replacing high-dose cytotoxic therapy with graft-versus-tumor effects, Blood 97 (2001) 3390.
7. MAIN, J.M., PREHN, R.T.: Successful skin homografts after the administration of high dosage X-radiation and homologous bone marrow, J Natl Cancer Inst 15 (1955) 1023.
8. MATHE, G., et al.: Adoptive immunotherapy of acute leukemia: Experimental and clinical results, Cancer Res 25 (1965) 1525.
9. NIEDERWIESER, D., et al. Allogeneic unrelated hematopoietic stem cell transplants (HSCT) after conditioning with 2 Gy total body irradiation (TBI), fludarabine (FLU) and a combination of cyclosporine (CSP) and mycophenolate mofetil (MMF) in patients ineligible for conventional transplants, Blood 96 (2000) Suppl 1:413a, #1778.
10. NOWELL, P.C., et al.: Growth and continued function of rat marrow cells in x-radiated mice, Cancer Res. 16 (1956) 258.
11. SANDMAIER, B.M., et al.: Nonmyeloablative conditioning for HLA-identical related allografts for hematologic malignancies, Blood 96 (2000) Suppl 1:479a, #2062.

12. STORB, R., *et al.*: Stable mixed hematopoietic chimerism in DLA-identical littermate dogs given sublethal total body irradiation before and pharmacological immunosuppression after marrow transplantation, Blood 89 (1997) 3048.
13. STORB, R., *et al.*: Stable mixed hematopoietic chimerism in dog leukocyte antigen-identical littermate dogs given lymph node irradiation before and pharmacologic immuno-suppression after marrow transplantation, Blood 94 (1999) 1131.
14. STORB, R., *et al.*: Stable mixed hematopoietic chimerism in dogs given donor antigen, CTLA4Ig, and 100 cGy total body irradiation before and pharmacologic immuno-suppression after marrow transplant, Blood 94 (1999) 2523.
15. STORB, R., *et al.*, Mixed chimerism after transplantation of allogeneic hematopoietic cells. In: E.D. Thomas, K.G. Blume, S.J. Forman (Eds.): Hematopoietic Cell Transplantation, 2nd Edition, Blackwell Science, Boston, (1999) 287–295.
16. STORB, R.,: Nonmyeloablative preparative regimens: experimental data and clinical practice. In: M.C. Perry (Ed.): ASCO Education Book, (1999) 241–249.
17. THOMAS, E.D., *et al.*: Bone-marrow transplantation, N Engl J Med 292 (1975) 832, 895.
18. WEIDEN, P.L., *et al.*: Antileukemic effect of graft-versus-host disease in human recipients of allogeneic-marrow grafts, N Engl J Med 300 (1979) 1068.
19. WEIDEN, P.L., *et al.*: Antileukemic effect of chronic graft-versus-host disease. Contribution to improved survival after allogeneic marrow transplantation, N Engl J Med 304 (1981) 1529.
20. YU, C., *et al.*: DLA-identical bone marrow grafts after low-dose total body irradiation: Effects of high-dose corticosteroids and cyclosporine on engraftment, Blood 86 (1995) 4376.

1.2 Allogeneic Stem Cell Transplantation after Reduced Conditioning in High-Risk Patients

Held[1], T. K., J. Schetelig[1], N. Kröger[2], C. Thiede[3], A. Krusch[1],
T. Zabelina[2], M. Dubiel[1], O. Rick[1], M. Bornhäuser[3], G. Ehninger[3],
A. R. Zander[2], W. Siegert[1]*

[1] Klinik für Innere Medizin mit Schwerpunkt Hämatologie und Onkologie, Charité –
Campus Virchow Klinikum, Berlin, [2] Knochenmarktransplantationszentrum,
Universitäts-Krankenhaus Eppendorf, Hamburg, [3] Medizinische Klinik und Poliklinik 1,
Universitätsklinikum Carl Gustav Carus, Dresden, Germany

* To whom correspondence should be addressed (wolfgang.siegert@charite.de)

Summary

We studied the toxicity and efficacy of reduced intensity conditioning followed
by allogeneic stem cell transplantation in 50 patients with an age of more than
50 years or with contraindications against myeloablative regimens. The
conditioning regimen consisted of fludarabine, busulphan, and rabbit anti-T-
lymphocyte globulin (ATG). Graft-versus-host disease (GvVHD) prophylaxis
was carried out with cyclosporine alone or in combination with methotrexate
or mycophenolate mofetil. Three graft failures occurred. GvHD-related
complications were a major cause of the 34% one-year, treatment-related,
mortality. Hence, the regimen itself can be carried out safely in high-risk
patients, but GvHD causes significant treatment-related mortality.

Introduction

In 1998, we adopted the protocol published by SLAVIN *et al.* [7] for patients
with an indication for allogeneic SCT but contraindications against the use of
a myeloablative regimen. We investigated whether the excellent tolerability as
reported by this group [7] could be reproduced in a larger group of patients
with an age of 50 years or more, with preceding autologous transplantation or
with significant co-morbidity.

Patients and methods

Between March 1998 and September 2000, 50 patients were treated at the
Charité – Campus Virchow Klinikum, Berlin or the Universitäts-Krankenhaus
Eppendorf, Hamburg. Median age was 50 years (range 20–64 years). Twenty-
six patients were male and 24 female. Diagnoses were chronic myeloid
leukaemia (n = 15), acute myeloid leukaemia (n = 9), myelodysplastic
syndromes (n = 9), malignant lymphoma (n = 11), refractory germ cell cancer
(n = 5) and breast cancer (n = 1). All patients had at least one contraindication
against a conventional myeloablative conditioning regimen. Twenty-seven
patients (54%) had two or more contraindications. Donors were 25 HLA-
identical siblings, 6 non-HLA-identical family members, 16 matched unrelated
donors and 3 unrelated donors with one minor mismatch.

The conditioning regimen consisted of fludarabine (180 mg/m²), busulphan (8 mg/kg) and rabbit ATG (40 mg/kg, Fresenius Inc.), as published [7]. Granulocyte colony-stimulating factor (G-CSF)-mobilized peripheral blood stem cells (PBSC) were transplanted in 36 patients. Fourteen patients with unrelated donors received bone marrow (BM). Supportive care as well as prophylaxis and treatment of infectious complications was carried out in a centre-specific manner. GvHD prophylaxis was carried out with CSA alone (n = 17), CSA plus short course methotrexate (MTX) (n = 18) or CSA plus mycophenolate mofetil (MMF) (n = 15). All data were computed with the SPSS statistical software (SPSS Inc., Chicago, Illinois). Kaplan-Meier product-limit estimates were used to analyse overall survival, treatment-related death and the cumulative incidence of GvHD. For the analysis of treatment-related death and of the incidence of GvHD, surviving patients and patients who died from relapse were censored at the day of last follow-up.

Results and discussion

Forty-seven patients were evaluable for engraftment, while three patients died before day +14. Neutrophil counts > 0.5/nl were reached after a median of 17 days (range 0–66) and platelet counts > 20/nl after 19 days (range 0–111). Until day +30, a median number of 9.5 red blood cell concentrates (range 0–24) and 6 single donor platelet apheresis concentrates (range 0–30) were given. Primary graft failure occurred in one patient with CML, who received bone marrow of a matched unrelated donor. We observed two secondary graft failures most likely due to CMV reactivation and subsequent treatment with ganciclovir. Between day 0 and day +30, patients had a median of 2 days (range 0–15) with fever of more than 38° C. Within the entire follow-up period, 9 patients died due to infectious complications at a median of 146 days (range 11–252) after transplantation. Acute GvHD grade II–IV was observed in 22 of 47 evaluable patients (47%) and acute GvHD grade III–IV in 5 patients (11%). Limited chronic GvHD was seen in 10 of 41 evaluable patients (24%), while 9 patients (22%) suffered from extensive GvHD. After a median observation period of 12 months (range 3–21), 22 patients are alive and 28 patients have died. Causes of death were disease progression in 14 patients and treatment-related complications in 14 patients. The actuarial 1-year overall survival is 40%. The 1-year probability of treatment-related mortality is 34%, including death due to GvHD.

During the last three years, several conditioning regimens with reduced dose intensity in conjunction with allogeneic stem cell transplantation have been studied [1]. Our aim was to reproduce the favourable data obtained in small-sized trials in a larger group of high-risk patients. Our data regarding engraftment and graft failure compare favourably to previously published results [4,5,7]. Severe infections during the first 30 days after transplantation were relatively rare and only one of our patients died from a lethal infection before day +30. Regarding the whole follow-up period, however, lethal infections occurred in 9 patients (18%) who were free from progression of their malignant disease. Apart from one patient, all of them suffered GvHD. Thus, the comparatively high incidence of lethal infections beyond the first month after transplantation is, presumably, the result of the high incidence and severity of acute and chronic GvHD.

Less tissue injury due to lower doses of cytotoxic agents in non-myeloablative regimens was assumed to reduce the incidence of GvHD. Further evidence for this assumption originates from experimental models where the induction of mixed chimerism prevented GvHD [8]. Considering our results and those from other groups, however, no empirical evidence indicates that reduced dose-intensity conditioning is associated with lower incidence and severity of GvHD [3,6]. Regarding survival, a 34% probability of treatment-related mortality at 1 year, including lethal complications of GvHD, compares with data obtained in aged patients [2].

In conclusion, the predominant problem using reduced conditioning was the occurrence of acute and chronic GvHD and the ensuing morbidity and mortality. In the context of a stimulation of tumour-specific T-cell activity, the induction of global alloreactivity could be beneficial.

Acknowledgements

We thank the staff of the Bone Marrow Transplantation Unit, Hamburg, for providing excellent patient care, and U. Löwel, M. Hartwig and P. Grassmel for excellent technical assistance in chimerism analysis. This work was supported in part by the Deutsche Krebshilfe (70-2755; CT).

References

1. CHAMPLIN, R., et al.: Harnessing Graft-versus-malignancy: non-myeloablative preparative regimens for allogeneic haematopoietic transplantation, an evolving strategy for adoptive immunotherapy. British Journal of Haematology 111 (2000) 18–29.
2. DEEG, H.J., et al.: Allogeneic and syngeneic marrow transplantation for myelodysplastic syndrome in patients 55 to 66 years of age. Blood 95 (2000) 1188–1194.
3. EHNINGER G., et al.: Dose-reduced conditioning for allografting in 45 patients with CML: a retrospective analysis. Blood 96 (2000) 783a.
4. NAGLER, A., et al.: Allogeneic peripheral blood stem cell transplantation using a fludarabine-based low intensity conditioning regimen for malignant lymphoma. Bone Marrow Transplantation 25 (2000) 1021–1028.
5. NIEDERWIESER, D., et al.: Allogeneic unrelated hematopoietic stem cell transplants after conditioning with 2 Gy TBI, Fludarabine and a combination of cyclosporine and mycophenolate mofetil in patients ineligible for conventional transplant. Blood 96 (2000) 413a.
6. SANDMAIER, B.M., et al.: Non-myeloablative conditioning for HLA-identical related allografts for hematologic malignancies. Blood 96 (2000) 479a.
7. SLAVIN, S., et al.: Non-myeloablative stem cell transplantation and cell therapy as an alternative to conventional bone marrow transplantation with lethal cytoreduction for the treatment of malignant and nonmalignant hematologic diseases. Blood 91 (1998) 756–763.
8. STORB, R., et al.: Stable mixed hematopoietic chimerism in DLA-identical littermate dogs given sublethal total body irradiation before and pharmacological immunosuppression after marrow transplantation. Blood 89 (1997) 3048–3054.

1.3 Non-Myeloablative Allogeneic Stem Cell Transplantation in Multiple Myeloma after Relapse: Low Transplant-Related Morbidity and Mortality

M. Görner*, L. Kordelas, M. Thalheimer, T. Luft, F. Ustaoglu, S. Pfeiffer, T. Moehler, M. Moos, H. Goldschmidt and A. D.Ho

Dept. of Haematology, Oncology and Rheumatology, University of Heidelberg, Heidelberg, Germany

* To whom correspondence should be addressed (martin_goerner@med.uni-heidelberg.de)

Summary

The existence of a graft-versus-myeloma effect has been well documented by responses to donor lymphocyte infusions and long-term survival following allogeneic bone marrow transplantation. The development of non-myeloablative conditioning regimens allows the utilization of allogeneic effects in patients usually not suitable for myeloablative allogeneic transplantation, i.e. older and heavily pretreated patients. In a small series of 13 patients with multiple myeloma who relapsed after one or two autologous transplantations, we show that conditioning with low-dose total body irradiation in combination with fludarabine allows stable engraftment and is well tolerated with low transplant-related morbidity and mortality. With a short median follow-up of 225 days, disease control was achieved only for patients in complete or partial remission after conventional treatment prior to allografting. Future studies have to define the role of non-myeloablative allogeneic transplantation as consolidation for patients responding to salvage therapy.

Introduction

Allogeneic bone marrow or peripheral stem cell transplantation have been reported to induce sustained and complete responses in multiple myeloma [3,5], but treatment-related morbidity and mortality usually are high and therefore only young patients received this treatment in the past [2]. Based on animal studies, various groups have recently developed different reduced intensity conditioning regimens, in order to minimize transplant-related toxicity [4,14], and first clinical trials have shown that mixed-haematopoietic chimerism can be achieved in patients using these non-myeloablative regimens [11,13,15].

In a monocentre pilot study, we tested whether allogeneic stem cell transplantation using reduced intensity conditioning can be performed as salvage therapy in heavily pretreated patients with multiple myeloma who relapsed after autologous transplantation. The objectives of the study were to evaluate safety and early engraftment.

Patients and methods

Patients

13 patients in whom myeloablative transplantation was contraindicated were conditioned with low-dose total body irradiation either alone or in combination with fludarabine. Patients received bone marrow (n = 1) or PBSC (n = 12) from either matched related (n = 4), mismatched related (n = 3) or unrelated donors (n = 6). All but one patient had chemosensitive relapse after one (n = 7) or two (n = 5) autologous transplantations. One patient with high-risk disease was unable to collect sufficient autologous stem cells and relapsed after multiple cycles of conventional chemotherapy. Characteristics of patients and donors are summarized in Table 1.3-1.

Preparative regimen

Eleven patients received fludarabine 30 mg/m^2 from day –3 to –1, and 2 Gy TBI at day 0 for conditioning followed by intensive immunosuppression post-transplant, using mycophenolate 2 x 15 mg/kg from day 0 to +28 and cyclosporine A from day –1 to +35 and were slowly tapered until day 100. CsA levels were aimed at 400 ng/ml until day +35. In two patients, only low-dose TBI was administered for conditioning.

Grafts

In 4 patients, at expected high risk for developing graft-versus-host disease, ex-vivo T-cell depletion of the G-CSF mobilized haematopoietic progenitors was performed using CD34 selection columns (Miltenyi), and 1 x 10^5/kg CD3 cells were added to the graft. 9 patients received unmanipulated grafts with a median content of 5 x 10^6 CD34$^+$ cells/kg BW.

Chimerism

Chimerism studies were performed by small tandem repeat amplification and analysis. PCR in bone marrow or peripheral blood samples was performed at days +28, +56 and +100, with the AmpFISTR Profiler PCR amplification kit (Applied Biosystems, Weiterstadt, Germany), and using the procedure recommended by the manufacturer. Separation and detection of the amplified

Table 1.3-1 Patient characteristics and disease status prior to allogeneic transplantation.

Number of patients	13
Median age at transplantation	52 (36–68)
Gender ratio	M:F = 10:3
Median time from diagnosis to transplantation	58 months (8–230)
Number of autologous transplantations prior to allogeneic transplantations	1 (n = 7) 2 (n = 5) 0 (n = 1)
Status prior to allogeneic transplantation	CR (n = 2) PR (n = 3) SD (n = 3) PD (n = 5)

PCR products was done on an ABI 310 automated sequencer (Applied Biosystems). The data were analysed with the Genescan 2.1 software (Applied Biosystems).

Definition of response

Complete remission (CR) was defined by 5% or less plasmocytes of normal morphology in the bone marrow and absence of monoclonal protein on serum electrophoresis and immunofixation analysis, and in case of Bence-Jones proteinuria by its disappearance. Partial response (PR) was defined by a decrease > 50% of paraprotein in serum, or > 90% in urine. Progression (PD) was defined as an increase > 25% of paraprotein, and patients not fulfilling either criteria for CR, PR or PD were, by definition, in stable disease (SD).

Results and discussion

Durable neutrophil and platelet engraftment of donor origin was observed in 11/13 patients. One patient, conditioned with only 2 Gy TBI, did not show allogeneic engraftment at all, was thereafter reconstituted with autologous cells, and is alive with a slowly progressive disease 550 days post transplant. In one other patient with rapidly progressing myeloma, who initially showed > 75% donor cells in the bone marrow, donor chimerism in the bone marrow decreased after one month, because disease progression was associated with > 90% plasma cell infiltration of the bone marrow.

A number of factors influence the engraftment of allogeneic stem cells, including the immunosuppressive properties of the conditioning regimen and the degree of HLA disparity between donor and recipient [1]. To be kept in mind: all patients in our series who received grafts of either related or unrelated, mismatched donors showed stable engraftment, suggesting that post-grafting immunosuppression was intense enough to permit engraftment across HLA barriers.

Conditioning therapy was very well tolerated. Only 46% of patients developed ANC < 0.5 x 10⁹/L, and platelet transfusions were required in only one patient (Table 1.3-2.). These results compare favourably with reports from studies in which a more intense, though not myeloablative conditioning was applied [12,7].

Table 1.3-2 Transplant-related morbidity and mortality.

GvHD 0–II	10/13 (77%)
GvHD III–IV	3/13 (23%)
Number of patients with ANC < 0.5 x 10⁹/L	6/13 (46%)
Number of patients with platelets < 50 x 10⁹/L	3/13 (23%)
Platelet transfusions (median number of units/pt)	0 (0–26)
Red blood cell transfusions (median number of units/pt)	2 (0–21)
CMV reactivation	3/13 (23%)
CMV disease	1/13 (8%)
Non-relapse mortality	0/13 (0%)

Table 1.3-3 Response to allogeneic transplantation.

Status prior to transplantation	Best response	Status at last follow-up
CR (n = 2)	CR (n = 5)	CR (n = 5)
PR (n = 3)	PR (n = 2)	PR (n = 0)
SD (n = 3)	SD (n = 2)	SD (n = 1)
PD (n = 5)	PD (n = 4)	PD (n = 7)*

CR = complete response, PR = partial response, SD = stable disease, PD = progressive disease
* 5/7 patients died at day +127, +137, +145, +317 and +486 because of progressive disease

Non-myeloablative conditioning regimens appear to be remarkably well tolerated in the early phase after transplantation, but they are associated with a significant risk of GvHD, which remains the major determinant of morbidity and mortality in patients with myeloma and other haematological malignancies, in which similar, standard myeloablative protocols are used [9,10]. In our series acute GvHD grade III–IV was diagnosed in 3/13 patients (23%), which compares favourably to other studies [6], in which an incidence of > 40% in a similar cohort of patients has been reported. In contrast to the study recently published by GARBAN *et al.*, post-grafting immunosuppression is more intense in our protocol, and given for a longer period, which may explain the low rate of acute GvHD. All our patients responded to steroids and mycophenolate, and no GvHD-related deaths occurred. Due to the short follow-up and the small number of patients, the incidence of chronic GvHD is difficult to assess from this study.

With the growing use of reduced intensity conditioning, several groups reported that infectious complications, in addition to GvHD, have an important impact on the outcome following non-myeloablative transplants [8,10]. This is supported by our analysis, since 3/13 (23%) patients showed CMV reactivation as documented by PCR and pp65-antigen. In all patients treatment with ganciclovir resulted in clearance of virus DNA. Symptomatic CMV-colitis developed in one patient with grade III GvHD.

In conclusion, the reduced intensity conditioning we used allows allogeneic stem cell transplantation as salvage therapy in heavily pretreated multiple myeloma patients, who relapse after autologous transplantation. With the protocol used, transplant-related morbidity and mortality were low, whereas lack of disease control emerged as the major problem. As shown in Table 1.3-3, especially patients in chemoresistant relapse progressed rapidly, and 5 out of 7 patients with progressive disease died, despite allogeneic transplantation. These preliminary results suggest that in the future, prior to allogeneic transplantation, a more aggressive conventional chemotherapy should be applied in order to achieve better disease control.

References

1. BACHAR-LUSTIG., E., *et al.*: Megadose of T cell-depleted bone marrow overcomes MHC barriers in sublethally irradiated mice. Nat Med 1 (1995) 1268–1273.
2. BENSINGER, W.I., *et al.*: Allogeneic marrow transplantation for multiple myeloma: an analysis of risk factors on outcome. Blood 88 (1996) 2787–2793.

3. BJORKSTRAND, B.B., *et al.*: Allogeneic bone marrow transplantation versus autologous stem cell transplantation in multiple myeloma: a retrospective case-matched study from the European Group for Blood and Marrow Transplantation. Blood 88 (1996) 4711–4718.

4. FUCHIMOTO, Y., *et al.*: Mixed chimerism and tolerance without whole body irradiation in a large animal model. J Clin Invest 105 (2000) 1779–1789.

5. GAHRTON, G., *et al.*: An update of prognostic factors for allogeneic bone marrow transplantation in multiple myeloma using matched sibling donors. European Group for Blood and Marrow Transplantation. Stem Cells 13 (1995) 122–125.

6. GARBAN, F., *et al.*: Immunotherapy by non-myeloablative allogeneic stem cell transplantation in multiple myeloma: results of a pilot study as salvage therapy after autologous transplantation. Leukemia 15 (2001) 642–646.

7. GIRALT, S., *et al.*: Engraftment of allogeneic hematopoietic progenitor cells with purine analog-containing chemotherapy: harnessing graft-versus-leukemia without myelo-ablative therapy. Blood 89 (1997) 4531–4536.

8. GIRALT, S., *et al.*: Non myeloablative "mini transplants". Cancer Treat Res 101 (1999) 97–108.

9. GOERNER, M., *et al.*: Allogeneic transplantation after lymphoablative conditioning in multiple myeloma. Bone Marrow Transplant 7 (suppl. 2) (2001) 247.

10. PORTER, D.L., *et al.*: Allogeneic cell therapy for patients who relapse after autologous stem cell transplantation. Biol Blood Marrow Transplant 7 (2001) 230–238.

11. SANDMAIER, B.M., *et al.*: Nonmyeloablative transplants: preclinical and clinical results. Semin Oncol 27 (2000) 78–81.

12. SLAVIN, S., *et al.*: Nonmyeloablative stem cell transplantation and cell therapy as an alternative to conventional bone marrow transplantation with lethal cytoreduction for the treatment of malignant and nonmalignant hematologic diseases. Blood 91 (1998) 756–63.

13. SLAVIN, S., *et al.*: Immunotherapy of hematologic malignancies and metastatic solid tumors in experimental animals and man. Bone Marrow Transplant 26 (Suppl. 2) (2000) 54–57.

14. STORB, R., *et al.*: Stable mixed hematopoietic chimerism in dog leukocyte antigen-identical littermate dogs given lymph node irradiation before and pharmacologic immuno-suppression after marrow transplantation. Blood 94 (1999) 1131–1136.

15. SYKES, M., *et al.*: Mixed lymphohaemopoietic chimerism and graft-versus-lymphoma effects after non-myeloablative therapy and HLA-mismatched bone-marrow transplantation. Lancet 353 (1999) 1755–1759.

1.4 Non-Myeloablative Allograft to Induce Graft-versus-Myeloma Effect after Cytoreductive Autotransplant for Multiple Myeloma

Kröger[1]*, N., R. Schwerdtfeger[2], W. Krüger[1], H. Renges[1], T. Zabelina[1], F. Tögel[1], N. Stute[1], G. Wittkowsky[2], R. Kuse[2], A. R. Zander[1]

[1] Bone Marrow Transplantation and Dept. of Haematology/Oncology, University Hospital, Hamburg, [2] Dept. of Haematology, A. K. St. Georg, Hamburg, Germany

* To whom correspondence should be addressed (nkroeger@uke.uni-hamburg.de)

Summary

In a pilot study, 8 patients with advanced stage II/III multiple myeloma and a median age of 48 years (range 32–63) received autografting after 200 mg/m^2 melphalan followed by a non-myeloablative regimen and allografting to induce a graft-versus-myeloma effect. The median interval between autologous and allogeneic transplantation was 89 days (range 60–139). The stem cell source was peripheral blood stem cells from either HLA-identical siblings (n = 5), siblings with one HLA-mismatch (n = 2) or from an HLA-compatible unrelated donor (n = 1). All patients engrafted and achieved 100% donor chimerism at a median of 30 days (range 19–38). One patient died on day +23 of infection (13%). Only one patient developed acute GvHD III. After a median follow-up of 12 months (range 5–14), 7 patients are alive without disease progression. Six (85%) are in CR with negative immunofixation, and one patient achieved PR with still decreasing monoclonal bands.

Introduction

Allogeneic stem cell transplantation is probably the only curative approach for patients with advanced multiple myeloma. Despite the high relapse rate, some patients survive long-term, free of disease after allogeneic transplantation [1]. The possible advantage of allogeneic stem cell transplantation is a proven graft-versus-myeloma effect by immunocompetent donor lymphocytes [6,12]. Despite better control of graft-versus-host disease and infectious complications, the treatment-related mortality of allogeneic transplantation is still between 17% and 40% [1,3,5,7], and therefore allogeneic transplantation remains only an option for young patients with HLA-identical siblings. Recently, so-called non-myeloablative regimens based on fludarabine or low-dose TBI have resulted in engraftment of allogeneic stem cells in patients with haematological diseases [4,8,11]. To reduce the treatment-related mortality, and to offer elderly patients with multiple myeloma the possibility of curative allogeneic transplantation, we developed a protocol consisting of high-dose chemotherapy supported by autologous stem cell transplantation, followed by a dose-reduced conditioning with allogeneic stem cell transplantation to induce a graft-versus-myeloma effect.

Table 1.4-1 Patients characteristics.

Patient/ Sex	Age	Stage	Prior therapy	Donor	Interval Auto-allotr. (days)	Source	Prior to auto	Prior to allo	After allo	L > 1.0	Plt > 20	RFLP (days)	aGvHD	Follow-up (days)
1. m.	32	IIIB	5x ID	MUD	102	PBSC	PR	CR	CR	15	14	Full (+20)	–	CCR 385+
2. m.	58	IIIA	4xID	Rel.-id	60	PBSC	PR	CR	CR	17	24	Full (+30)	–	CCR 378+
3. m.	48	IIA	4x MP, 5xID	Rel.-mm	103	PBSC	PR	PR	CR	15	20	Full (+20)	Skin I	Died +22 after allo (Sepsis/pneumonia)
4. m.	63	IIA	4xVAD	Rel.-id	84	PBSC	MR	PR	CR	16	16	Full (+38)	–	CCR 371+
5. m.	49	IIIB	3xMP, 3x VCAP	Rel.-mm	77	PBSC	PR	PR	CR	16	26	Full (+36)	Skin / gut III	CCR 361+
6. m.	44	IIA	3xVAD/ 1xCyclo.	Rel.-id	94	PBSC	PR	CR	CR.	20	23	Full (+30)	Gut I	CCR 273+
7. f.	48	IIIA	4xID	Rel.-id	119	PBSC	MR	PR	PR*	17	33	Full (+20)	–	PR *256+
8. m.	53	IIIA	3xVCAP/ 1xCycl.	Rel.-id	135	PBSC	PR	PR	CR	18	26	Full (+24)	Too early	CCR 225+

* currently still decreasing monoclonal bands

ID = idarubicin/dexamethason, MP = melphalan/prednisone, VCAP = oncovertin, cyclophosphamide, adriamycin, prednisone, VAD = oncovertin, adriamycin, dexamethasone

Rel-id = HLA-identical sibling, MUD = matched unrelated donor, mm = mismatched, PBSC = peripheral blood progenitor cell, CCR = continuous complete remission

Patients and methods

Between 10/1999 and 12/2000, 14 patients were enrolled in the protocol. In 12/2000, 8 patients had completed autologous and allogeneic transplantation and were evaluable for toxicity and response. The median age was 48 years (range 32–63). There were 7 male and one female patients. All patients had advanced disease (stage II/III) and at least minor response after anthracycline-containing induction chemotherapy. The median β2-microglobulin was 2.6 mg/dl (range 1.0–3.5). Two patients responded to therapy with anthracycline after failing to respond to melphalan/prednisone therapy. After stem cell mobilization with cyclophosphamide (4 g/m²) or G-CSF alone from steady state haematopoiesis, patients received high-dose melphalan (200 mg/m²) followed by autologous stem cell support. After an interval of 3 months, patients received a dose-reduced conditioning, consisting of melphalan 100 mg/m², fludarabine 180 mg/m² and anti-thymocyte globulin (rabbit, Fresenius, Bad Homburg, Germany) given at a dose of 10 mg/kg over 12 hours on days –3, –2 and –1, followed by allogeneic stem cell transplantation on day 0. In case of incomplete chimerism or persistent disease, additional donor lymphocyte infusions were planned. All patients received peripheral blood stem cells from either HLA-identical siblings (n = 5), siblings with one HLA mismatch (n = 2) or from an HLA-compatible unrelated donor (n = 1). GvHD prophylaxis consisted of cyclosporine A (3 mg/kg, given from day –1 to three months post transplantation. Cyclosporine A was tapered from day 75 and discontinued on day 100. Methotrexate (10 mg/m²) was given on day 1, 3 and 6 post transplantation.

   Chimerism was verified by PCR analysis of tandem repeat sequences of hypervariable DNA regions. The standard criteria were used for acute and chronic GvHD [10]. The study was approved by the local Ethics Committee. Patient characteristics are given in Table 1.4-1.

Results and discussion

The median transplanted CD34+ cell number for autologous transplantation was 5.8 x 10⁶/kg BW (range 2.2–10.9 10⁶/kg BW). A leukocyte count of > 1000/mm³ was achieved after a median of 12 days (range: 11–13) and of platelet > 20000/mm³ after a median of 14 days (range 13–25). The median interval between autologous and allogeneic transplantation was 89 days (range 60–135). No mortality after autologous transplantation was observed, and 3/8 (38%) achieved a complete remission. After dose-reduced allogeneic transplantation, engraftment was observed in all patients with leukocyte engraftment (> 1000/mm³) after a median of 16 days (range 15–20), and platelet engraftment (> 20000/mm³) after a median of 24 days (range 14–33). Complete donor chimerism was detected in all patients after a median of 30 days (range 19–38). After allogeneic transplantation 6 of 7 achieved CR (85%) according to EBMT criteria, with negative immunofixation, and one patient with PR has still decreasing monoclonal bands. One patient died with multiorgan failure after sepsis and pneumonia on day 22 after allogeneic transplantation, resulting in a treatment-related mortality of 13%. Three of the six evaluable patients did not experience acute GvHD. Two patients experienced mild acute GvHD grade I and one patient (17%) with mismatch transplantation had grade III GvHD of the skin and gut.

After a median follow-up of 12 months (range 5–14) after autologous transplantation, and 8 months (range 3–11) after allogeneic transplantation, 7 out of 8 patients (88%) are alive without disease progression. This preliminary data demonstrate that a dose-reduced conditioning regimen with allogeneic transplantation, after prior cytoreduction with autologous stem cell transplantation, is a feasible and highly effective approach, even in elderly patients with a high rate of complete remission.

The possibility of dose-reduced or non-myeloablative conditioning to minimize transplant-related mortality and achieve at least mixed chimerism with preservation of a graft-versus-leukaemia effect has been recently described [4,8,11]. The concept of tumour debulking by autologous stem cell transplantation, preceding a non-myeloablative regimen with allografting, was used by CARELLA in 15 patients with malignant lymphoma [1]. In his study, all patients engrafted, and 87% had 100% donor chimerism. 11 of the 15 patients achieved a CR after the combined procedures, while nearly 50% experienced grade II or higher acute GvHD, and two developed extensive chronic GvHD. In our melphalan-based and dose-reduced regimen (100 mg/m²), no graft failure was observed and all patients experienced a rapid and complete donor chimerism. The preceding autologous transplantation may have induced significant host immunosuppression, which should contribute to rapid and full donor engraftment after allotransplantation. We noted a high proportion of complete remission (85%) after allografting. In two patients, CR was achieved after three months post allografting, suggesting a delayed anti-myeloma effect. We observed a low incidence of severe GvHD, especially in HLA-compatible donors. In a similar study in patients with myeloma, the Seattle group [9] used autografting after melphalan, 200 mg/m², followed by a low dose TBI (2 Gy) regimen with allografting to induce a graft-versus-myeloma effect. Six out of 12 achieved a CR. The incidence of grade II GvHD was 50% and two patients died of grade IV GvHD. Because of the delayed graft-versus-myeloma effect a more cytotoxic conditioning regimen than low-dose TBI may be advisable, especially in patients with risk of early relapse. Our preliminary data of the auto-allotransplant-protocol with a complete response rate of 85% and a treatment-related mortality of 13% are encouraging; however, a longer follow-up is needed to determine both late mortality and curative potential in comparison to conventional allografting in patients with multiple myeloma.

Acknowledgements

We thank the staff of the BMT unit for providing excellent care of our patients and the medical technicians for their excellent work in the BMT laboratory.

This work was supported by a grant of the Roggenbuck-Stiftung.

References

1. BJÖRKSTRAND, B., *et al.*: Allogeneic bone marrow transplantation versus autologous stem cell transplantation in multiple myeloma: a retrospective case-matched study from the European Group for Blood and Marrow Transplantation. Blood 88 (1996) 4711–4718.
2. CARELLA, A.M., *et al.*: Autografting followed by nonmyeloablative immunosuppressive chemotherapy and allogeneic peripheral blood haematopoietic stem cell transplantation as treatment of resistant Hodgkin's disease and Non-Hodgkin's lymphoma. J Clin Oncol 18 (2000) 3918–3924.
3. GAHRTON, G., *et al.*: Progress in allogeneic haematopoietic stem cell transplantation for multiple myeloma. Bone Marrow Transplant. 2000 25 (Suppl 1): 140.
4. GIRALT, S., *et al.*: Engraftment of allogeneic haematopoietic progenitor cells with purin analog-containing chemotherapy: Harnessing graft-versus-leukemia effect without myeloablative therapy. Blood 89 (1997) 4531–4536.
5. KRÖGER, N., *et al.*: Allografting in advanced multiple myeloma with anti thymocyte globulin to prevent graft-versus-host disease. (submitted)
6. LOKHORST, H.M., *et al.*: Donor lymphocyte infusion for relapsed multiple myeloma after allogeneic stem cell transplantation: predictive factors for response and long-term outcome. J Clin Oncol 18 (2000) 3031–3037.
7. MAJOLINO, I., *et al.*: Allogeneic transplantation of unmanipulated peripheral blood stem cells in patients with multiple myeloma. Bone Marrow Transplant 22 (1998) 449–455.
8. McSWEENEY, P., STORB, R. Establishing mixed chimerism with immunosuppressive, minimally myelosuppressive conditioning: Preclinical and clinical studies. American Society of Haematology Educational Book (1999) 396–405.
9. MOLINA, A., *et al.*: Non-myeloablative peripheral blood stem cell allografts following cytoreductive autotransplants for treatment of multiple myeloma . Blood 96 (Suppl) (2000) 2063.
10. PRZEPIORKA, K.M., *et al.*: 1994 Consensus Conference on acute GvHD-grading. Bone Marrow Transplant 15 (1995) 825–828.
11. SLAVIN, S., *et al.*: Nonmyeloablative stem cell transplantation and cell therapy as an alternative to conventional bone marrow transplantation with lethal cytoreduction for the treatment of malignant and nonmalignant diseases. Blood 91 (1998) 756–763.
12. TRICOT, G., *et al.*: Graft-versus-myeloma effect: proof of a principle. Blood 87 (1996) 1196–1198.

1.5 Non-Myeloablative Blood Stem Cell Transplantation for Patients with Haematologic Malignancies and Poor Prognosis

Kobbe[1]*, G., P. Schneider[1], D. Schubert[1], F. Zohren[1], M. Aivado[1],
R. Fenk[1], H. Pape[2], R. Kronenwett[1], F. Neumann[1], R. Haas[1]

[1] Dept. of Haematology, Heinrich Heine University, Düsseldorf, [2] Dept. of Radiotherapy,
Heinrich Heine University, Düsseldorf, Germany

*To whom correspondence should be addressed (Kobbe@med.uni-duesseldorf.de)

Summary

To induce graft-versus-tumour reactions without the side effects of an intensive myeloablative conditioning regimen 22 patients with advanced haematologic malignancies and contraindications for a conventional allogeneic transplantation received mobilized blood stem cells from HLA-identical related or unrelated donors after treatment with Fludarabine (3×30 mg/m^2) and low-dose TBI. Patients were treated either during steady state haematopoiesis or in the cytopenic phase of a preceding chemotherapy. After transplantation, sequential analysis of chimerism and minimal residual disease were performed on selected cell populations from blood and bone marrow.

Twenty patients (90%) engrafted. Of 14 evaluable patients with active disease, 8 had responses. In 5 patients a remission was achieved with 2 patients with multiple myeloma in partial remission, 2 patients with chronic myeloid leukaemia in molecular remission and 1 high grade non-Hodgkin's lymphoma in complete remission. Of 5 patients who were transplanted in remission, 4 are disease-free (2 patients with MDS, 1 patient with Hodgkin's disease and 1 patient with non-Hodgkin's lymphoma). Eight patients died, of which 7 of disease progression and 1 of treatment-related complications (treatment-related mortality: 5.3%). Twelve out of 18 evaluable patients (67%) have developed acute GvHD (6x II°, 6x III°–IV°), and five out of 10 patients alive beyond day 100 have chronic GvHD (extensive: 2, limited: 3). Our data demonstrate that non-myeloablative blood stem cell transplantation is well tolerated and is able to induce remissions in a variety of haematologic cancers.

Introduction

For decades, allogeneic blood stem cell transplantation has relied on intensive myeloablative conditioning regimens to cure malignant disease, genetic defects of haematopoiesis and autoimmune disorders [1]. Although postulated early, it was only at the beginning of the 1990s that scientists began to acknowledge that allogeneic graft-versus-leukaemia reactions contribute much to the cures observed after allogeneic blood stem cell transplantation [2,5,7]. The graft-versus-malignancy reaction following allogeneic stem cell transplantation involves donor immune effector cells and is capable of inducing molecular remissions in several haematologic malignancies. During the last few years increasing effort has been spent on transplantation techniques that are less toxic but allow the engraftment of allogeneic haematopoietic stem cells [4,6,8,11,13]. We have used such a minimal myelosuppressive conditioning regimen in a series of patients with advanced haematologic malignancies and contraindications to a conventional myeloablative conditioning regimen.

Material and methods

Patients and donors

Twenty-two patients (median age 47 years, range 39–64) with haematologic malignancies received a non-myeloablative conditioning regimen followed by allogeneic blood stem cell transplantation either during steady state haematopoiesis (n = 19) or in the cytopenic phase of a preceding chemotherapy course (n = 3). The diagnosis were acute myeloid leukaemia (3), myelodysplastic syndrome (4), chronic myeloid leukaemia (4), non-Hodgkin's lymphoma (4), Hodgkin's disease (1) and multiple myeloma (6). Thirteen of the 22 patients were in an advanced phase of their disease and 8 patients had already received an autologous blood stem cell transplantation. All except 3 patients with chronic myeloid leukaemia had contraindications or high-risk characteristics for a conventional allogeneic stem cell transplantation.

HLA-identical sibling donors received G-CSF (Neupogen 12,5 µg/kg, Amgen, Munich) as a single daily subcutaneous injection. Large-volume leukapheresis was begun at day 5 and continued until a total of 5 x 10^6 CD34$^+$ cells/kg were harvested. If possible, larger numbers of CD34$^+$cells were obtained. HLA-identical unrelated donors were treated according to the protocol of the providing centre. All apheresis products were infused on the apheresis days without further storage or manipulation.

Conditioning regimen and supportive care

All patients received fludarabine, 30 mg/m^2, day –4 until day –2 (Fludarabine, Medac, Munich, Germany). On day –1, oral or intravenous medication with Cyclosporine A, target trough levels 300–350 ng/ml (Sandimmun optoral, Novartis, Nuremberg, Germany) was initiated. On day 0, patients received a single dose of 200 cGy total body irradiation followed by the infusion of the allogeneic apheresis product. On the evening of that day additional immunosuppression with mycophenolate mofetil, 2 x 1.5 mg/kg (Cellcept, Roche, Grenzach-Whylen, Germany) was initiated and continued until day 28. Prophylactic antibiotic and antifungal therapy was given when neutrophil levels fell below 500/µl. Patients with a positive serology for CMV or a CMV-positive donor received oral ganciclovir, 3 x 0.5 g (Cymeven oral, Roche, Grenzach-Whylen, Germany) beginning on day 28. The remaining patients received antiviral prophylaxis with famiciclovir, 2 x 250 mg (Famvir zoster, SmithKline Beecham, Munich, Germany). In addition, all individuals received PCP prophylaxis with trimetoprim and sulfamethoxazol, 1 x twice a week (Bactrim forte, Roche, Grenzach-Whylen, Germany). Patients were treated on an outpatient basis where possible.

Chimerism analysis and quantification of minimal residual disease

We performed sequential chimerism testing of defined cell populations by means of STR (short tandem repeat) PCR. The following four polymorphic loci were used: TPOX, HUMTH01, CSF1PO, and HUMAR. After magnetic cell selection (Milteniyi Biotec, Bergisch Gladbach, Germany) and DNA extraction a total of 150 ng DNA was subjected to PCR containing fluorescence labelled primers. Amplicons were detected by automated DNA fragment analysis on a 6% polyacrylamide gel in a DNA A.L.F.-express II sequencer (Amersham Pharmacia Biotech, Freiburg, Germany). The fluorescent gel data were calculated using ALF Win Fragment Analyzer 1.02 software.

Minimal residual disease was monitored with molecular techniques using the Light Cycler technology (Roche Diagnostics, Mannheim, Germany) where possible. For t(9;22) the Light Cycler real time RT-PCR can detect and quantify fusion transcripts resulting from the breakpoints b3a2, b2a2, b2a3, b3a3 and e1a2. Detection of G6PDH and BCR-ABL-PCR products was performed by measuring fluorescence using a specific pair of hybridization probes. Normalization against a standard of the housekeeping gene G6PDH was used to correct for differences in BCR-ABL and G6PDH values resulting from different quality of RNA isolation, cDNA synthesis and PCR. This serial dilution standard of known G6PDH concentration allowed quantification of BCR-ABL transcripts in blood and bone marrow.

Results

Toxicity and engraftment

The applied treatment regimen was well tolerated. Non-haematologic side effects were rare and included nausea and vomiting following total body irradiation as well as one case of WHO grade III renal toxicity and one case of WHO grade III hepatic toxicity. Cytopenia was mild with a median minimal white blood count of 1,000/μl (range 100–4,900) and a minimal median platelet count of 40,000/μl (range 2,000–247,000). The 3 patients who were transplanted in the cytopenic phase of a preceding chemotherapy course recovered a white blood count greater than 1,000/μl after a median of 9 days (range 8–17) and a platelet count of greater than 50,000/μl after a median of 13 days (range 12–30). One patient developed late pure red cell aplasia which finally resolved after treatment with erythropoietin, mycophenolate mofetil and high-dose immunoglobulin. All patients had evidence of donor cell engraftment at day 14. Twenty patients recovered normal blood counts with increasing donor cell chimerism. One patient with advanced CML transformed into blast crisis at day 20 and 1 patient with MDS, myelofibrosis and severe cytopenia never reached normal blood counts until she died on day 65 despite a constant donor chimerism of about 30%. Both patients were classified as graft failures. Following initial engraftment 6 (3 AML, 2 CML, 1 MDS) out of 20 patients had declining donor chimerism in blood or bone marrow because of increasing numbers of malignant recipient cells.

Graft-versus-host disease

Acute graft-versus-host disease greater than grade II developed in 12 out of 19 (67%) evaluable patients. GvHD occurred spontaneously in 9 and after donor lymphocyte infusion in 3 patients. In 10 patients acute GvHD resolved after treatment while two patients had refractory aGvHD. Both patients died, 1 of progressive lymphoma and the other of a myocardial infarction. Five of 11 patients, alive beyond day 100, suffer from chronic GvHD (3 limited, 2 extensive). Both patients with extensive chronic GvHD received transplants from matched unrelated donors.

Response and survival

Among the 14 evaluable patients with active disease at the time of transplantation, 8 had responses, which were only transient in 3. In five individuals a remission was achieved with 2 patients with multiple myeloma in partial remission, 2 patients with chronic myeloid leukaemia in molecular remission, and one patient with non-Hodgkin's lymphoma in complete remission. Details on two of these patients are outlined in Figures 1.5-1 and 1.5-2. All patients achieving remission had 100% donor chimerism. Of the 5 patients who were treated in remission (2 MDS, 2 NHL, 1 HD) only one patient with a non-Hodgkin's lymphoma relapsed and died of disease progression. The remaining 4 patients are alive in complete remission with 100% donor haematopoiesis.

After a median follow-up of 130 days (range 50–586), 8 patients died at a median of 106 days after transplantation (range 50–129). Seven patients died

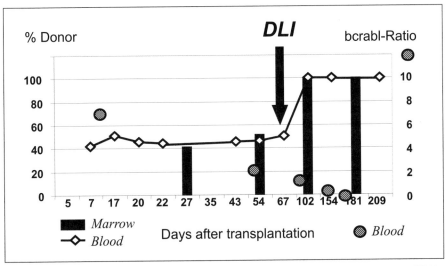

Figure 1.5-1 A 53-year-old man with CML in first chronic phase received 8.19 x 10⁶ CD34⁺ cells/kg from his HLA-identical brother after conditioning with fludarabine and low-dose TBI. Following transplantation, he developed mixed chimerism with about 50% donor cells in blood and marrow. On day 67, he was given 1 x 10⁷ CD3⁺ cells/kg from his donor. About 4 weeks later, he presented with acute GvHD III° and converted to full donor chimerism. PCR for bcr-abl became negative. He now is alive at day +577, in molecular remission, without signs of chronic GvHD.

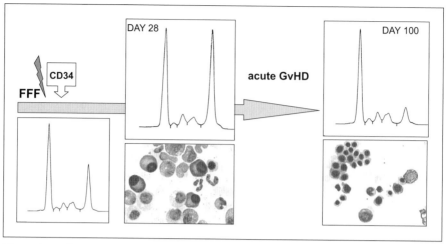

Figure 1.5-2 A 45-year-old man with multiple myeloma, IgG kappa, who was in refractory relapse after 2 autotransplants and after treatment with thalidomide received 6.1 x 10⁶ CD34⁺ cells from a matched unrelated donor after conditioning with fludarabine and low- dose TBI. After transplantation, he developed full donor chimerism but experienced further disease progression. Following cessation of the prophylactic immunosuppression, he developed acute GvHD III° and an excellent response of the myeloma. The paraprotein decreased rapidly and malignant plasma cells were cleared from the bone marrow. He now is alive at day 130+, in very good partial remission on immunosuppressive treatment for chronic GvHD.

of disease progression, and one from myocardial infarction (treatment-related mortality 5.3%).

Discussion

Our data demonstrate that a minimal intensive conditioning regimen consisting of fludarabine and low-dose TBI exerts minimal toxicity in patients with haematologic malignancies and advanced age or comorbid conditions. The observed treatment-related mortality of about 5% in a group of high-risk patients compares favourably with the mortality of conventional myeloablative conditioning regimens [9]. Despite low toxicity, engraftment was achieved in the great majority of patients, confirming earlier studies by STORB and colleagues [11].

We observed impressive responses, especially in patients with multiple myeloma, chronic myeloid leukaemia and non-Hodgkin's lymphoma. Disease response was usually seen in conjunction with the development of acute GvHD. Unfortunately, some patients displayed progressive disease despite acute GvHD. All 3 individuals with advanced acute myeloid leukaemia who were not in remission at the time of transplantation had no benefit from the procedure. In these patients disease progression was unchanged by repeated donor lymphocyte infusions.

These findings are in line with experiences of others groups using dose-reduced conditioning regimens in high-risk patients. CHILDS *et al.* demonstrated the curative potential of non-myeloablative blood stem cell transplantation for patients with CML in 1999, and SANDMAIER *et al.* recently reported a 67% molecular response rate in patients with CML treated with a similar low intensity conditioning regimen [3,10]. BADROS *et al.* observed a clinical response in 12 out of 16 (75%) patients with advanced multiple myeloma transplanted after conditioning with an intermediate dose of melphalan (100 mg/m^2) [1]. In their series too, response was closely linked to the development of acute GvHD, which contributed to a treatment-related mortality of 18%.

Grafts-versus-host disease caused significant morbidity in our group of patients as more than 60% developed acute GvHD of grade II or greater, and 50% of patients surviving more than 100 days developed chronic GvHD. Extensive chronic GvHD may be especially a problem in the case of matched unrelated donor transplantation. Future studies will have to focus on reducing GvHD severity without losing the benefits of allogeneic graft-versus-malignancy reactions. Up to now, there are no accurate tests or prognostic factors to predict which patient's disease will ultimately respond to an allogeneic graft-versus-malignancy reaction. It is therefore essential to accumulate further experience in various haematologic malignancies and solid tumours to identify patient groups that will have the greatest benefit of this new transplantation modality.

References

1. BADROS, A., *et al.*: High response rate in refractory and poor-risk multiple myeloma after allotransplantation using a nonmyeloablative conditioning regimen and donor lymphocyte infusions. Blood 97 (2001) 2574.
2. BARNES, D.W.H., *et al*: Treatment of murine leukemia with x-rays and homologous bone marrow: preleminary communication. Br Med J 2 (1956) 626.
3. CHILDS, R., *et al.*: Molecular remission of chronic myeloid leukemia following a nonmyeloablative allogeneic peripheral blood stem cell transplant: in vivo and in vitro evidence for a graft-versus-leukemia effect. Br J Haematol, 107 (1999) 396.
4. GIRALT, S., *et al.*: Engraftment of allogeneic hematopoietic progenitor cells with purine analo-containing chemotherapy: Harnessing graft-versus-leukemia without myeloablative therapy. Blood 89 (1997) 4531.
5. HOROWITZ, M.M., *et al*: Graft-versus-leukemia reactions after bone marrow transplantation. Blood 75 (1990) 555.
6. KHOURI, I.F., *et al.*: Transplant lite: Induction of graft-versus-malignancy using fludarabine-based nnonablative chemotherapy and allogeneic blood progenitor-cell transplantation as treatment for lymphoid malignancies. J Clin Oncol 16 (1998) 2817.
7. KOLB, H.J., *et al*: Donor leukocyte transfusions for treatment of recurrent chronic myeloid leukemia in marrow transplant patients. Blood 76 (1990) 2462.
8. MCSWEENY, P.A., *et al.*: Outpatient PBSC allografts using immunosuppression with low-dose TBI before, and cyclosporine (CSP) and mycophenolate mofetil (MMF) after transplant. Blood 92 (1998) Suppl.1: 519a.
9. PETERSEN, F.B. and BEARMAN, S.I.: Preparative regimens and their toxicity. In: Thomas ED, Blume KG, Forman SJ (Eds.). Bone Marrow Transplantation. Blackwell Science, 1994.
10. SANDMAIER, B.M., *et al*: Induction of molecular remissions in chronic myelogenous leukemia (CML) with nonmyeloablative HLA-identical sibling allografts. Blood 96 (2000) Suppl. 1: 861a.
11. STORB, R., *et al.*: Mixed Chimerism after transplantation of allogeneic hematopoietic cells. In: Thomas ED, Blume KG, Forman SJ (eds). Hematopoietic Cell Transplantation (ed2) Boston, MA, Blackwell Science (1999) 287.

12. THOMAS, E.D., *et al.*: Bone marrow transplantation (First of two parts). N Engl J Med 277 (1975) 832.
13. YU, C., *et al.*: Synergism between mycophenolate mofetil and cyclosporine in preventing graft-versus-host disease among lethally irradiated dogs given DLA-nonidentical unrelated marrow grafts. Blood 91 (1998) 2581.

1.6 Preliminary Results of Allogeneic Stem Cell Transplantation after Reduced Conditioning in Chronic Lymphocytic Leukaemia

Schetelig[1], J., T. K. Held[1], M. Bornhäuser[2], C. Thiede[2], G. Ehninger[2], M. Kiehl[3], A. A. Fauser[3], R. Schwerdtfeger[4], N. Kröger[5], A. Zander[5], J. Beyer[6], A. Neubauer[6], W. Siegert[1]*

[1]Charité, Campus Virchow Klinikum, 11. Medizinische Klinik, Schwerpunkt Hämatologie und Onkologie, Berlin, [2]Carl-Gustav-Carus-Universität, Dresden, [3]Klinik für Knochenmarktransplantation, Idar-Oberstein, [4]Deutsche Klinik für Diagnostik, Wiesbaden, [5]Universitäts-Krankenhaus Eppendorf, Hamburg, [6]Hämatologie, Klinikum der Philipps-Universität, Marburg, Germany

* To whom correspondence should be addressed (wolfgang.siegert@charite.de)

Summary

The aim of this study was to assess whether haematopoietic cell transplantation (HCT) after dose-reduced conditioning is feasible and effective in patients with CLL. For this purpose, 20 patients with a median age of 50 years (range 34–62) and a median of 3 preceding chemotherapy regimens received HCT after a conditioning regimen with fludarabine, busulphan and anti-T-lymphocyte globulin (ATG). Donors were 9 HLA-identical siblings, one non-HLA-identical related donor and 10 matched unrelated donors.

Results

Chemotherapy was well tolerated with mild mucositis and acceptable liver or renal toxicity. Acute GvHD II°/III°/IV° was observed in 7/3/1 patients, respectively. Limited chronic GvHD occurred in 7 patients and extensive disease in 4 patients. After a median follow-up of 12 months (range 3–28), 18 patients are alive. One patient died of acute GvHD IV° and one of progressive disease. Nine patients reached partial remissions. 10 patients reached complete immunological remissions and became negative for CD5/CD19 co-expressing cells in peripheral blood after a median of 3 months (range 1–10).

Conclusions

After dose-reduced HCT in CLL we observed a high remission rate. Treatment-related mortality was low, but GvHD caused significant morbidity. Remissions as late as 10 months after HCT can be interpreted as a graft-versus-lymphoma effect in CLL.

Introduction

Chronic lymphocytic leukaemia is not curable with conventional chemotherapy, and the average survival in patients who relapse after first-line treatment is 24 months [2]. Forty percent of the patients are younger than 60 years and 10% are younger than 50 years at the time of diagnosis. Especially for these patients, new therapeutic approaches with a curative attempt are warranted. Allogeneic HCT has been performed in some patients with advanced disease in small-sized studies or on an individual basis [3,4,5]. About 40% of the patients achieved long- term disease-free survival, which argues in favour of an immunologic effect against B-CLL. However, the fact that about 40% of the patients died treatment-related had a significant impact on overall survival [4].

In 1998, SLAVIN and colleagues demonstrated that a dose-reduced conditioning regimen consisting of fludarabine, busulphan and ATG provided enough immunosuppression to prevent graft rejection [6]. Without cytotoxic eradication of host haematopoiesis, stable chimerism developed and subsequently the eradication of malignant cells was observed. There is hope that with this new approach allogeneic immunotherapy could be applied without extensive treatment-related mortality [1]. These results prompted us to study whether HCT after dose-reduced conditioning is feasible and effective in CLL patients.

Patients and methods

Patients and donors

In our study, 20 patients with B-CLL were treated between July 1998 and July 2000 in six German bone marrow transplantation centres. Median age was 50 years (range 34–62). Seven patients were of female sex and 13 were males. The median duration from first diagnosis to HCT was 3.8 years, and a median number of 3 chemotherapy regimens had been applied before HCT. Donors were 9 HLA-identical siblings, 1 non-HLA-identical related donor and 10 matched unrelated donors.

Transplantation procedure

The conditioning regimen consisted of fludarabine (180 mg/m²), busulphan (8 mg/kg) and rabbit ATG (40 mg/kg, Fresenius Inc.) as published by SLAVIN in 1998 [6]. Granulocyte colony-stimulating factor-mobilized peripheral blood stem cells (PBSC) were transplanted in 18 patients. The median count of CD34-positive cells in PBSC products was 6.4×10^6 CD34+ cells/kg (range 3.0–12.6 x 10^6). Two patients with unrelated donors received bone marrow with 1.3 and 1.4×10^8 mononuclear cells/kg. GvHD prophylaxis consisted of cyclosporine monotherapy or in combination with "short course" MTX or MMF.

Results

Engraftment

Neutrophil counts of more than 0.5/nl were reached after a median of 17 days (range 11–40). Platelet counts of more than 20/nl were reached after a median of 13 days (range 0–34). A median of 3 (range 0–24) single donor platelet apheresis concentrates and a median of 8 (range 0–21) units of red blood cells were transfused. Two patients needed no platelet or red blood cell support. No primary graft failure, but one secondary graft failure occurred.

Toxicity and GvHD

Patients had a median of 1.5 days with fever and 12 patients suffered from infections requiring intravenous antibiotics. Chemotherapy was well tolerated with mild mucositis and acceptable liver (4x CTC II° and 1x CTC III°) or renal toxicity (2x CTC II°). Acute GvHD II°/III°/IV° was observed in 7/3/1 patients respectively. Chronic GvHD occurred in 11 of 18 evaluable patients (7x limited, 4x extensive disease).

Response and survival

Nine patients are in partial remission according to NCI criteria. A complete immunological remission defined as negativity for CD5/CD19 co-expressing cells was observed in 10 patients. These patients became negative for CD5/CD19 co-expressing cells in peripheral blood after a median of 3 months (range 1–10). After a median follow-up of 12 months (range 3–28), 18 patients were alive, two patients had died. One patient died of acute GvHD IV° and one patient from progressive disease.

Discussion

Our response data indicate that allogeneic stem cell transplantation after dose-reduced conditioning can induce complete remissions even in patients with advanced disease. The fact that remissions occurred as late as ten months after transplantation argues strongly in favour of a graft-versus-leukaemia effect. So far only one patient had progressive disease. However, a longer follow-up will be needed in order to assess the quality of the remissions.

Chemotherapy-associated toxicity is acceptable. Nevertheless acute and chronic GvHD causes significant morbidity. Incidence and severity of GvHD are within the range one would expect after classic allogeneic transplantation. Treatment-related mortality is relatively low compared to conventional allogeneic transplantation [4,5]. However, the low number of patients restricts conclusions about the applicability of dose-reduced allogeneic stem cell transplantation in the course of this indolent malignoma.

In conclusion, we observed a high remission rate in patients with CLL after a dose-reduced conditioning regimen and HCT. There is good evidence of a graft-versus-leukaemia effect in CLL. Treatment-related mortality was low, but acute and chronic GvHD caused significant morbidity. The observed extent of GvHD argues in favour of a more intensive prevention of GvHD. However, one has to be aware that the intensification of immunosuppression might weaken the graft-versus-leukaemia effect. Therefore it is essential to come to a better understanding of the mechanisms of the graft-versus-leukaemia effect. It would be most desirable to learn how to stimulate tumour-specific T-cell reactivity instead of the induction of global alloreactivity.

References

1. CHAMPLIN, R., et al.: Harnessing Graft-versus-malignancy: non-myeloablative preparative regimens for allogeneic haematopoietic transplantation, an evolving strategy for adoptive immunotherapy. Br J Haematol 111 (2000) 18.

2. KEATING, M. J., *et al.*: Long-term follow-up of patients with chronic lymphocytic leukemia receiving fludarabine regimens as initial therapy. Blood 92 (1998) 1165.
3. KHOURI, I. F., *et al.*: Autologous and allogeneic bone marrow transplantation for chronic lymphocytic leukemia: preliminary results. J Clin Oncol 12 (1994) 748.
4. MICHALLET, M., *et al.*: Allogeneic haematopoietic stem cell transplantation for chronic lymphocytic leukemia: results and prognostic factors for survival after transplantation. Analysis from EBMT registry. Blood (2000) 205a (Abstract).
5. PAVLETIC, Z. S., *et al.*: Outcome of allogeneic stem cell transplantation for B cell chronic lymphocytic leukemia. Bone Marrow Transplant 25 (2000) 717.
6. SLAVIN, S., *et al.*: Non-myeloablative stem cell transplantation and cell therapy as an alternative to conventional bone marrow transplantation with lethal cytoreduction for the treatment of malignant and nonmalignant hematologic diseases. Blood 91 (1998) 756.

Part Two
Related and Unrelated Donors
in Allogeneic Stem Cell Transplantation

2.1 Review of Allogeneic Transplantation in Multiple Myeloma

Gösta Gahrton

Depts. of Medicine and Haematology, Huddinge University Hospital, Stockholm, Sweden

Summary

Allogeneic bone marrow transplantation for multiple myeloma has been performed in younger patients since 1982. Since 1994, results of matched sibling donor transplants have improved due to lower transplant-related mortality. The overall 4-year survival is now more than 50 per cent. Important favourable prognostic factors are to be a female, to have received few pre-transplant treatment regimens, and to be responsive to treatment. There is no significant difference in outcome using bone marrow or peripheral blood stem cells.

Molecular remission can be obtained in about 40% of patients and is associated with reduced relapse rate. Non-myeloablative transplant regimens may well reduce transplant-related mortality further, and the use of donor lymphocyte transfusions may play a role in reducing relapse rate and/or may induce remissions in relapsed disease.

Introduction and early studies

Attempts to treat patients with multiple myeloma with allogeneic bone marrow transplantation (BMT) were made already in the early 1980s [10,17,25,28]. At Huddinge University Hospital, the first patient received a transplant in 1983 [10]. The patient had had the disease for many years but became refractory to treatment. An allogeneic transplant was performed with a matched sibling donor and the patient went into complete remission. She stayed in complete remission without symptoms for four years, and we thought that she was the first patient with multiple myeloma that had been cured from the disease. However, shortly thereafter, she relapsed but lived as a mixed chimera for another six years, when she died from progression of the disease.

In 1987, results of a series of 14 patients transplanted at centres reporting to the European Group for Blood and Marrow Transplantation (EBMT) registries were published [11]. At the time of follow-up, 10 patients had survived for 6–34 months following transplantation, and 5 were well and in complete haematologic remission.

From now on, selected younger patients with multiple myeloma underwent BMT throughout the world. In 1991, the EBMT reported 90 patients that had undergone BMT with marrow from HLA-matched sibling donors [12]. The complete remission rate was 43 per cent of all patients, and 58 per cent of those who could be evaluated. The optimism was great, since there was a seemingly plateau-like survival curve at 40 per cent from 36 to 76 months. All but one of the 12 patients at risk on the plateau were still in complete haematologic remission.

Prognostic factors were delineated in this [12] and later EBMT studies [13,14]. The most important favourable pre-transplant ones were: to be a female, to have received only one line of treatment, and to be in complete remission at the time of transplantation. Other factors that tended to be of importance were: to be in stage I at the time of diagnosis and to have low serum beta-2-microglobulin levels at diagnosis. The most important favourable post-transplant factor was to enter a complete remission. Those patients had a highly significant better survival than those who did not enter a complete remission. A post transplant predictor of very poor survival was to have severe graft-versus-host disease grades III and IV. Such patients, although few, usually succumbed within months.

Most centres within the EBMT used total body irradiation, 10–12 Gy, fractionated or unfractionated, with lung shielding + cyclophosphamide, 60 mg/kg x 2, for conditioning. The Seattle Group presented results of a series of patients conditioned with busulphan + cyclophosphamide (BuCy) [6,7]. Most of the patients received busulphan 14–16 mg/kg + cyclophosphamide 60 mg/kg x 2. Transplant-related mortality was high with the higher dosages, but otherwise the results seemed comparable to EBMT results.

High-dose treatment followed by autologous transplantation (ABMT) was performed at many centres in parallel with BMT in another or the same centres [2,3,4,23,26]. Initially, transplant-related mortality was significant with ABMT also, although considerably lower than with BMT. In an attempt to compare BMT and ABMT, a case-matched study was performed utilizing patient data in the EBMT registry [5]. This study showed that transplant-related mortality was significantly higher with BMT, while the relapse rate of patients who entered a complete remission was lower with BMT than with ABMT. However, the lower relapse rate could not compensate for the higher transplant-related mortality, and the overall survival was poorer with BMT than with ABMT. However, the study also showed that the difference in outcome was mainly due to a poorer survival with BMT in male patients, while there was no significant difference between BMT and ABMT in female patients. Thus, to be a female patient was a favourable prognostic factor for BMT but not for ABMT.

Recent studies

Since 1995, results of BMT in multiple myeloma have improved [15]. The EBMT group was able to show that there had been significant improvement in overall survival and transplant-related mortality in patients who had received a matched sibling donor transplant from 1994 to 1998 as compared to those who had received a transplant before that time (1983–1993). The overall 4-year survival in 334 patients who received BMT during the latter time period was only 35 per cent, as compared to 55 per cent in 223 patients who received BMT from 1994 to 1998. There was no significant difference in survival between the patients who had received bone marrow for transplantation during this later time period and those 133 patients who had received allogeneic peripheral blood stem cells. The reason for the lower transplant-related mortality was probably a combination of factors, *i.e.* patients were receiving the transplant earlier and therefore had received fewer pre-transplant treatment regimens.

Also, there were fewer deaths due to bacterial and fungal infections and interstitial pneumonitis. Thus, probably more effective supportive care and the use of new more effective antibacterial, antifungal and antiviral drugs also played a role.

Since 1995, allogeneic peripheral stem-cell transplants had been given to an increasing number of patients. However, an early belief that transplantation with peripheral blood stem cells may have caused the lower overall transplant-related mortality during the later time period could not be proven. Peripheral blood stem cell transplants were not superior, and did not tend to be superior to transplants with bone marrow during the same time period. Chronic graft-versus-host disease, after peripheral blood stem cells graft, was more frequent than after bone marrow transplantation, but there appeared to be no clear difference in acute graft-versus-host disease. As for relapse rate, it was too early to judge, but the tendency was towards no difference between those BMT that had been performed before 1994 and those which had been performed later. Also, there was no trend towards a difference in relapse rate between peripheral blood stem cell transplants and BMT performed during the same time period from 1994 to 1998.

CORRADINE et al. [9] have shown that molecular remissions, using patient specific oligonucleotides from the CDR2 and CDR3 regions of the immuno-globulin, can be obtained in a fraction of patients following allogeneic transplantation. Out of 14 investigated patients, 7 obtained a molecular remission. On the other hand, only one out of 15 patients who received an autologous transplant, entered molecular remission, which was of short duration. A recent expansion of the allogeneic group of patients to 42 showed that 17 (40 per cent) obtained a molecular remission. Associated with the molecular remission was a significantly lower haematological relapse rate, which was also superior to the rate obtained after haematological remission [8].

Donor lymphocyte transfusions and non-myeloablative transplantation

Since the discovery that donor lymphocyte transfusion could induce remissions in other haematological disorders as well [19], this approach has also been successful in multiple myeloma [1,21,22,29]. These studies showed that it was possible to obtain a remission , following relapse, in a fraction of patients (probably less than 30 per cent) after donor lymphocyte transfusions. The results seemed to indicate that intensive regimens may not be necessary in order to induce remissions in multiple myeloma. Instead, one could perhaps take advantage of a graft-versus-leukaemia effect. Therefore, non-myeloablative regimens, as previously described for other haematological disorders [27], were attempted by several groups. Encouraging results have been obtained using a variety of regimens. Some of these regimens are not clearly non-myeloablative, but dosages are lower than those usually used in allogeneic transplantation. MOLINA and co-workers used a regimen of pre-transplant conditioning with a total body irradiation dosage of no more than 200 cGy [24]. In the early trials, the regimen was not combined with further immunosuppressive conditioning, but was followed by cyclosporine and mycophenolate mofetil post transplant, in order to prevent graft-versus-host disease. Later on, total body irradiation at the same dose was combined with fludarabine for conditioning. The most promising results were obtained when the non-myeloablative transplant followed ABMT.

Other regimens used were combinations of melphalan + fludarabine [16] or melphalan + fludarabine + CAMPATH-1H [18]. Here, too, engraftment was obtained in the majority of cases, and remissions also occurred.

Recently, LALANCETTE et al. [20] collected data on 54 patients who had received a non-myeloablative transplant at EBMT centres. A variety of regimens were used for conditioning, but most patients received melphalan plus fludarabine. GvHD prophylaxis also varied. Cyclosporine + ATG/ALG was mostly utilized (n = 26), followed by cyclosporine and T-cell depletion (n = 17). Only one patient was in complete remission and 29 in partial remission before the transplant, while 18 had refractory or relapsed disease. After transplant, 19 patients were in complete remission while only 12 still had refractory disease. Encouraging was that good-risk patients had only 13 per cent transplant-related mortality, and 83 per cent one-year survival. Poor-risk patients, however, showed high transplant-related mortality (68 per cent) and poor survival (25 per cent).

The EBMT group has recently started a prospective study in which non-myeloablative allogeneic transplantation with sibling donors will be performed prior to ABMT, in comparison to ABMT alone. The conditioning regimen includes total body irradiation with 200cGy + fludarabine 30 mg/kg for 3 days and GvHD prevention with cyclosporine + mycophenolate mofetil. Hopefully, this regimen will reduce both transplant-related mortality as compared to BMT and relapse rate as compared to ABMT.

References

1. ASCHAN J., et al.: B. LONNQVIST, O. RINGDEN, G. KUMLIEN, G. GAHRTON: Graft-versus-myeloma effect [letter; comment]. Lancet 348 (1996) 346.
2. ATTAL, M., et al.: A prospective, randomized trial of autologous bone marrow transplantation and chemotherapy in multiple myeloma. Intergroupe Français du Myelome [see comments]. N Engl J Med 335 (1996) 91–97.
3. BARLOGIE, B., et al.: High-dose melphalan with autologous bone marrow transplantation for multiple myeloma. Blood. 67 (1986) 1298–1301.
4. BJORKSTRAND, B., et al.: Prognostic factors in autologous stem cell transplantation for multiple myeloma: an EBMT Registry Study. European Group for Bone Marrow Transplantation. Leuk Lymphoma;15 (1994) 265–272.
5. BJORKSTRAND, B., et al.: Allogeneic bone marrow transplantation versus autologous stem cell transplantation in multiple myeloma: a retrospective case-matched study from the European Group for Blood and Marrow Transplantation. Blood 88 (1996) 4711–4718.
6. BENSINGER W.I., et al.: Allogeneic marrow transplantation for multiple myeloma: an analysis of risk factors on outcome. Blood 88 (1996) 2787–2793.
7. BENSINGER, W.I., et al.: Phase I study of busulfan and cyclophosphamide in preparation for allogeneic marrow transplant for patients with multiple myeloma. J Clin Oncol 10 (1992) 1492–1497.
8. CORRADINI, P., et al.: Molecular remissions are frequently achieved in myeloma patients undergoing allografting with peripheral blood stem cells. Bone Marrow Transplantation 27 (Suppl 1) (2001) 39.

9. CORRADINI P., *et al*: Molecular and clinical remissions in multiple myeloma: role of autologous and allogeneic transplantation of hematopoietic cells. J Clin Oncol 17 (1999) 208–215.

10. GAHRTON, G., *et al*.: Bone marrow transplantation in three patients with multiple myeloma. Acta Med Scand 219 (1986) 523–527.

11. GAHRTON, G., *et al*.: Bone marrow transplantation in multiple myeloma: report from the European Cooperative Group for Bone Marrow Transplantation. Blood 69 (1987) 1262–1264.

12. GAHRTON, *et al*.: Allogeneic bone marrow transplantation in multiple myeloma using HLA-compatible sibling donors – an EBMT Registry Study. Bone Marrow Transplant 7 (Suppl 2) (1991) 32.

13. GAHRTON, G., *et al*.: An update of prognostic factors for allogeneic bone marrow transplantation in multiple myeloma using matched sibling donors. European Group for Blood and Marrow Transplantation. Stem Cells 13 (Suppl. 2) (1995) 122–125.

14. GAHRTON, G., *et al*.: Prognostic factors in allogeneic bone marrow transplantation for multiple myeloma [see comments]. J Clin Oncol 13 (1995) 1312–1322.

15. GAHRTON, G., *et al*.: Progress in allogeneic bone marrow and peripheral blood stem cell transplantation for multiple myeloma: a comparison between transplants performed 1983-1993 and 1994-1998 at the European Group for Blood and Marrow Transplantation Centres. Br J Haematol 113 (2001) 209–216.

16. GIRALT, S., *et al*.: Non-Myeloablative conditioning with Fludarabine/Melphalan (FM) for patients with multiple myeloma (MM). Blood 994 (Suppl. 1) (1999) 347a, Abstract 1549.

17. HIGHBY, D.B., *et al*.: Bone marrow transplantation in multiple myeloma: a case report with protein studies. In: ASCO proceedings, 1982 (1982) p. C747.

18. KOTTARIDIS, P.D., *et al*.: In vivo CAMPATH-1H prevents graft-versus-host disease following nonmyeloablative stem cell transplantation. Blood 96 (2000) 2419-2425.

19. KOLB, H.J., *et al*.: Graft-versus-leukemia effect of donor lymphocyte transfusions in marrow grafted patients. European Group for Blood and Marrow Transplantation Working Party Chronic Leukemia. Blood 86 (1995) 2041–2050.

20. LALANCETTE, M., *et al*.: Excellent outcome of non-myeloablative stem cell transplant (NMSCT) for good-risk myeloma: The EBMT experience. Blood 96 (2000) 204a.

21. LOKHORST, H.M., *et al*.: Donor lymphocyte infusions for relapsed multiple myeloma after allogeneic stem-cell transplantation: predictive factors for response and long-term outcome. J Clin Oncol 18 (2000) 3031–3037.

22. LOKHORST, H.M., *et al*.: Donor leukocyte infusions are effective in relapsed multiple myeloma after allogeneic bone marrow transplantation. Blood 90 (1997) 4206–4211.

23. McELWAIN, T.J., R.L. POWLES: High-dose intravenous melphalan for plasma-cell leukaemia and myeloma. Lancet 2 (1983) 822–824.

24. MOLINA, A., *et al*.: Non-myeloablative peripheral blood stem cell (PBSC) allografts following cytoreductive autotransplants for treatment of multiple myeloma (MM). Blood (1999) 94 (Suppl. 1) 347a, Abstract 1551.

25. OZER, H., *et al*.: Allogeneic BMT and idiotypic monitoring in multiple myeloma. In: AACR abstracts; 1984 (1984) 161.

26. SELBY, P., *et al*.: The development of high-dose melphalan and of autologous bone marrow transplantation in the treatment of multiple myeloma: Royal Marsden and St Bartholomew's Hospital studies. Hematol Oncol 6 (1988) 173–179.

27. SLAVIN, S., *et al*.: Nonmyeloablative stem cell transplantation and cell therapy as an alternative to conventional bone marrow transplantation with lethal cytoreduction for the treatment of malignant and nonmalignant hematologic diseases. Blood 91 (1998) 756–763.

28. TURA, S., *et al*.: Bone marrow transplantation in multiple myeloma. Scand J Haematol 36 (1986) 176–179.

29. TRICOT, G., *et al*.: Graft-versus-myeloma Effect: proof of principle. Blood 87 (1996) 1196–1198.

2.2 Allogeneic Stem Cell Transplantation from Related and Unrelated Donors for Active Leukaemia or Lymphoma: Feasibility and Results in Elderly Patients

Finke, J., K. Potthoff, S. Mielke, H. Bertz

Abteilung Hämatologie & Onkologie, Medizinische Universitätsklinik, Freiburg, Germany

Summary

Elderly patients (> 60 y) with AML or myelodysplasia have a dismal prognosis with chemotherapy alone. Furthermore, age greater than 60 years is a generally accepted exclusion criterion for allogeneic transplantation as the only curative treatment for these diseases. Here we report our experience with a novel dose-intensity-reduced regimen. The median age was 63 years (range 61–70). 22 patients were transplanted with PBSC (n = 20) or BM (n = 2) from HLA-matched related (n = 8) or unrelated (n = 14) donors. Diagnoses were AML/MDS (18), MPS (1), CLL (2), RCC (1). Except for 3 patients in CR1 or CR2, all other patients had active malignant disease, the majority with excessive marrow infiltration, either refractory, relapsing or untreated. Pre-transplant conditioning was performed with fludarabine 5×30 mg/m^2 in combination with BCNU 2×150 mg/m^2, melphalan 110 mg/m^2 (FBM). For GvHD prophylaxis cyclosporine A plus mini-Mtx or mycophenolate mofetil was used. In cases of unrelated-donor-derived grafts, patients received ATG-S (Fresenius) prior to transplant. Acute GvHD > °II occurred in 5 patients. 5 patients died due to relapse (1) or infection (4). With a median follow-up time of 180 days, projected 1-year disease-free survival is 75%. These results compare favourably with data obtained in younger patients with similar advanced diseases treated with high-dose regimen, where we achieved a 1-year DFS of 74% (n = 35) after unrelated donor PBSCT and 32% 1-year DFS (n = 62) after unrelated donor BMT. Thus, allogeneic PBSCT combined with novel fludarabine/melphalan-based regimen is well suitable for elderly patients with advanced haematologic malignancies resulting in high CR rates after related as well as unrelated donor transplantation. Patients with a high risk for relapse or not reaching CR should rapidly be referred to allogeneic stem cell transplantation; with our regimen the upper age limit can be extended to about 70 years. Our and others' data suggest that compared to BMT, PBSCT results in better survival rates in advanced disease patients.

Introduction

Allogeneic stem cell transplantation presents the only chance of cure in the majority of elderly patients with acute leukaemia or myelodysplasia. Due to the toxicities of high-dose chemo-/radiotherapy conditioning, and a higher incidence of severe acute graft-versus-host disease in the elderly patient, the upper age limit of 50 to 55 years has been generally accepted in allogeneic transplantation until recently. The acknowledgement of the importance of the graft-versus-leukaemia/malignancy effect for long-term cure has initiated several approaches with reduced doses of chemo- or radiotherapy. Successful engraftment as well as the induction of complete remission has been shown with immunosuppressive conditioning alone [1,2,4,6,7,8].

Previously, we established a regimen with reduced intensity conditioning consisting of fludarabine as lymphotoxic agent in combination with alkylating agents [9]. The rationale was to enable engraftment of stem cells from related as well as unrelated donors and to apply moderate doses of cytotoxic agents with broad activity but negligible heart, lung, bladder or gastrointestinal toxicity as well as good CNS penetration and easy i.v. application, aiming for practicability in the elderly or in patients with coexisting disease. The action of both BCNU and melphalan is not influenced by the cell cycle; they are thus able to destroy proliferating as well as resting "dormant" malignant cells. Here we describe a successful allogeneic stem cell transplantation in elderly patients with active leukaemia.

Patients and methods

A total of 22 patients aged 61 to 70.5 years (median 63.6) with AML (4), AML secondary to MDS (11), MDS RAEBt or CMML (2), MDS RA (1), OMF (1), CLL (2) and renal cell cancer (1) were included in this study. Prior to transplantation 1 patient was in CR, 2 were in CR2/CP2 , and 5 patients were untreated, 6 in relapsing and 8 with primary refractory disease. The advanced state of disease is further illustrated by the bone marrow blast counts in the 18 patients with AML/MDS: the degree of bone marrow infiltration was $> 15–30\%$ in 4 patients, and exceeded 30 to $> 90\%$ in 10 patients. For conditioning, patients received fludarabine 30 mg/m^2/day from day –9 to day –5, BCNU 150 mg/m^2/day at day –7 and –6, and melphalan 110 mg/m^2 at day –4 (FBM protocol) [9]. For GvHD prophylaxis, cyclosporine A was started at day –3 in combination with methotrexate in the first 2 patients, which was then replaced by mycophenolate mofetil in the following patients. Rabbit anti-T-lymphocyte globulin (20 mg/kg/day) (ATG-S, Fresenius, Bad Homburg, Germany) was given at day –2 and day –1 in the cases of unrelated donor transplantation [5], except for one patient with platelet antibodies, thus refractory to platelet transfusion. Marrow (n = 2) or peripheral blood (n = 20) stem cell grafts were obtained from related (n = 8) or unrelated (n = 14) HLA-identical donors. Standard inpatient supportive care was given as described and G-CSF (filgrastim) was given from day +7 onwards.

Results and discussion

Median time to leukocyte engraftment (WBC $> 1000/\mu l$) was day +11, and platelet engraftment ($> 20\ 000/\mu l$ and $50\ 000/\mu l$) was day +16 and +18 respectively.

Acute graft-versus-host disease °II–°IV developed in 11 patients. Three patients died from fungal infection that had been active during the previous course of leukaemia treatment, and one patient died from sepsis and MOF secondary to acute GvHD, resulting in a treatment-related mortality of 18%. Nineteen of the total of 22 patients reached a CR, 1 patient had stable disease and 2 patients were not evaluable owing to death after early infection. Four patients relapsed and one patient died due to relapse. With a median follow-up time of 6 months, projected 1 year overall and progression-free survival is 75% and 60%, respectively. No difference was observed between patients transplanted from matched siblings or matched unrelated donors.

The results obtained in this patient group with very old and advanced disease compare well to data from our standard adult (age 18 to 56 years) allogeneic transplant program. The standard allogeneic transplant recipient up to 56 years of age is conditioned using high-dose busulfan/cyclophosphamide for myeloid malignancies, or 12 Gy TBI in combination with cyclophosphamide and VP-16 for lymphoblastic leukaemia. Here we were able to improve the outcome considerably in our unrelated donor transplant group due to novel preventive measures against GvHD by the use of *in-vivo* T-lymphocyte modulation with ATG [5]. Standard GvHD prophylaxis consists of cyclosporine A and short course methotrexate and in the case of matched or mismatched unrelated donor transplantation additional ATG is given.

Patients are grouped according to stage of disease, the "early disease group" with patients in first CR of acute leukaemia or first chronic phase in CML, and the "advanced disease group" for the remainder, comprising only a few CR2 cases and patients primarily refractory to treatment as well as relapsed or untreated patients. In the early disease group the disease-free survival after 4 years is 77% for both matched related (n = 109) and unrelated (n = 43) transplantation. In the advanced disease group overall survival at 4 years is 39% for 96 unrelated donor transplants and 35% for 132 matched sibling transplants. Recently, we repeatedly succeeded in obtaining G-CSF-mobilized peripheral blood-derived grafts for unrelated donor transplantation. Within the advanced disease group, and with grafts from unrelated donors, we observed an overall survival of 74% in 35 patients transplanted with PBSC and 32% in 62 patients transplanted with bone marrow. Despite the shorter follow-up time in the PBSCT group as compared to the BMT group, the difference is statistically significant. A longer follow-up time period is necessary to further establish the role of PBSCT in unrelated donor transplantation.

The results, however, are promising, and although we cannot completely exclude improvements in supportive care and in patient management in the future, we attribute the better results to the higher number of stem cells and T-cells and, possibly, antigen presenting cells in PBSC grafts. This will contribute to a better graft-versus-leukaemia effect; moreover, a more polyclonal haemato-poiesis is likely to confer a better resistance to infection or other proliferative impairment of the lympho-haematopoietic system in the recipient. Our findings are in line with a recent randomized trial comparing PBSC with BM in matched sibling donor transplantation [3]. We would further infer that the addition of ATG prior to unrelated-donor transplantation allows a faster reduction of cyclosporine A, thus reducing long-term immunosuppression and the risk of subsequent relapse.

In conclusion, the novel FBM regimen is well tolerated in patients beyond age 60. The regimen is highly active in advanced leukaemia, resulting in complete remission in the majority of patients. Treatment-related mortality correlates with the pre-transplant performance status and a history of aspergillosis. With our GvHD prevention strategy, results from unrelated donors equal those obtained from matched sibling donors. The use of PBSC seems to confer an advantage regarding survival in advanced leukaemia patients.

Finally, age or active leukaemia are not exclusion criteria for allogeneic transplantation. Therefore, early HLA typing and a rapid start in donor-search is recommended in patients with acute, high-risk leukaemia or MDS. A careful selection of reduced intensity regimen and the differential application of graft sources as well as post-transplant monitoring of minimal residual disease and chimerism will further improve long-term survival and allow for the application of allogeneic transplantation where necessity prevails.

References

1. BARRETT, A. J.: Non-myeloablative stem cell transplants. Br J Haematol 111 (2000) 6.
2. BARRETT, A. J. AND R. CHILDS: The benefits of an alloresponse: Graft-versus-tumor (review). J Hematotherapy & Stem Cell Research 9 (2001) 347.
3. BENSINGER ,W. I., et al.: Transplantation of bone marrow as compared with peripheral-blood cells from HLA-identical relatives in patients with hematologic cancers. New Engl J Med 344 (2000) 175.
4. CHILDS, R., et al.: Regression of metastatic renal-cell carcinoma after nonmyeloablative allogeneic peripheral-blood stem-cell transplantation. New Engl J Med 343 (2000) 750.
5. FINKE, J., et al.: Allogeneic bone marrow transplantation from unrelated donors using in vivo anti-T cell globulin. Br J Haematol 111 (2000) 303.
6. GIRALT, S., et al.: Melphalan and purine analog-containing preparative regimens: reduced-intensity conditioning for patients with hematologic malignancies undergoing allogeneic progenitor cell transplantation. Blood 97 (2001) 631.
7. NAGLER, A., et al.: Allogeneic peripheral blood stem cell transplantation using a fludarabine-based low-intensity conditioning regimen for malignant lymphoma. Bone Marrow Transplantation 25 (2000) 1021.
8. SANDMAIER, B. M., et al.: Nonmyeloablative conditioning for HLA-identical related allografts for hematologic malignancies. Blood 96 (2000) 479a.
9. WÄSCH, R., et al.: Rapid achievement of complete donor chimerism and low regimen-related toxicity after reduced conditioning with fludarabine, carmustine, melphalan and allogeneic transplantation. Bone Marrow Transplantation 26 (2000) 243.

2.3 Reduced Toxicity on Conditioning with Treosulfan and Fludarabine

Casper[1]*, J., W. Knauf[2], U. Hammer[3], H. Wegener[3], B. Steiner[1], D. Wolf[1], A. Knopp[1], H.-D. Kleine[1], M. Freund[1]

[1] Dept. of Haematology and Oncology, University of Rostock, Rostock,
[2] Dept. of Haematology and Oncology, Klinikum Benjamin Franklin, FU Berlin, Berlin,
[3] Dept. of Forensic Medicine, University of Rostock, Rostock, Germany

*To whom correspondence should be addressed (jochen.casper@med.uni-rostock.de)

Summary

Treosulfan and fludarabine, applied as conditioning agents for allogeneic blood stem cell transplantation, have been used in a phase I/II study. Twenty-five patients, otherwise non-eligible for allogeneic transplantation, with a median age of 50 years have been transplanted with CML, AML, MDS, multiple myeloma, NHL cbcc and CLL. Ten matched related donors (MRD), 1 mismatched related donor and 14 matched unrelated donors (MUD) donated bone marrow or peripheral blood stem cells. Conditioning consisted of treosulfan 10 g/m^2 i.v. d –6 to d –4 and fludarabine 30 mg/m^2 i.v. d –6 to d –2. Patients with unrelated donors received, in addition, ATG (rabbit) 10 mg/kg d –4 to d –2. Besides ATG in MUD transplantation cyclosporine A was given as GvHD prophylaxis only. Leukocyte recovery > 0.5 Gpt/l and > 1 Gpt/l occurred by median day +9 (range 0–18) and day +10 (range 0–19), respectively. Platelet recovery (> 50 Gpt/l) occurred by median day +15 (range 8 to not reached). Extra-medullary toxicity was mild, not exceeding CTC °II, except for ALAT/ASAT elevation in 5, and bilirubine in 1 patient (maximum °III). However, three of these 5 patients had started the conditioning therapy with increased liver enzymes. Additionally, in one patient, a peripheral polyneuropathy occurred (CTC °III) – this patient had been heavily pre-treated, and the cause of this polyneuropathy remains still unclear. Complete chimerism was reached among 20 of 23 patients by day +28 (2 too early). One patient had a primary graft failure, and recovered with his own haematopoiesis. The donor chimerism of the other two patients is still increasing. Complete donor chimerism has been maintained by all patients except for 2 patients with CML. Both became Philadelphia positive again, but could be cured by reduction of the immune suppression or repeated DLI. The treatment-related mortality after a median observation time of 233 days is 4/25 patients. One additional patient with multiple myeloma died, due to complications of his concurrent cardiac amyloidosis. With an overall survival of 80% and a failure-free survival of 68%, the further evaluation of the treosulfan and fludarabine combination may lead to a promising toxicity-reduced conditioning regimen with sufficient stem cell toxicity, immuno-suppression and anti-leukaemic activity.

Introduction

Toxicity-reduced and/or non-myeloablative conditioning regimen may expand the patient population who may benefit from allogeneic transplantation [1,2,7]. Several different approaches are currently under investigation with fludarabine being a major component in many of them [3]. We combined fludarabine with treosulfan.

Treosulfan, a structural analogue of busulfan, is an alkylating agent with pronounced effect against committed as well as early haematopoietic stem cells [4]. Besides an intravenous mode of application, treosulfan is non-enzymatically activated to the alkylating mono- and diepoxides under physiologic conditions (pH 7.4). In a phase I study with autologous blood stem cell transplantation, a maximum tolerable dose of 47 g/m^2 was determined without any non-haematologic side effects exceeding II° CTC [6].

For allogeneic transplantation in a phase I/II study, we choose a cumulative treosulfan dose of 30 g/m^2, corresponding to two thirds of the maximum tolerated dose, in combination with fludarabine.

Methods

Twenty-five patients were transplanted using the treosulfan/fludarabine conditioning regimen. They were either heavily pre-treated (7 with previous autologous or allogeneic transplantation), aged > 49 years (n = 13; median age 50 years, range 20–60) or/and had severe concomitant diseases (n = 9). Ten matched related and 14 unrelated, as well as one mismatch-related donor contributed peripheral blood stem cells (n = 15) or bone marrow (n = 10). A median number of 2.3 x 10^6 CD34$^+$ cells/kg bodyweight of the recipient (range 0.39–15.9) were used for transplantation.

Indications for transplantation were CML (6), MDS (4), AML 6 (incl. 2 secondary AML), multiple myeloma (4) (including 2 with severe amyloidosis), NHL cbcc (3) and CLL (2). A median follow-up of 233 days (range 1–590) has been reached.

Treosulfan 10 g/m^2 i.v. was given from d –6 to d –4, fludarabine 30 mg/m^2 i.v. from d –6 to d –2. In addition, patients with unrelated donors received ATG (rabbit) 10 mg/kg from d –4 to d –2. Besides ATG in MUD transplantation, cyclosporine A was given solely as GvHD prophylaxis.

Results

Treosulfan/fludarabine conditioning was well tolerated. The leukocyte nadir occurred on day +5 (median 0.44 Gpt/l) remaining above 0.5 Gpt/l in 6/25 patients (Figure 2.3-1). Leukocyte recovery > 0.5 Gpt/l and > 1 Gpt/l occurred by median day +9 (range 0–18) and day +10 (range 0–19), respectively. The leukocyte depression was of short duration with a median of 4 days below 0.5 Gpt/l (range 0–13) and < 1 Gpt/l of 8 days (range 0–15). Platelet recovery (>50 Gpt/l) occurred by median day +15 (range 8 to not reached) (Figure 2.3-2).

Extra-medullary toxicity was mild, not exceeding CTC °II except for ALAT/ASAT increase in 5 and bilirubine in 1 out of 25 patients (maximum °III).

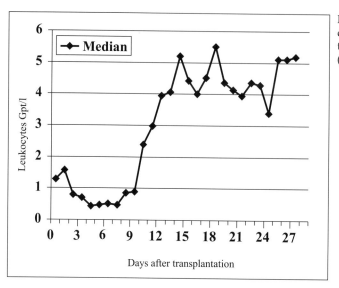

Figure 2.3-1 Leukocyte counts after transplantation (median values).

However, three of these 6 patients had started the conditioning therapy with a pre-existing liver enzyme elevation. Additionally, in one patient, a peripheral polyneuropathy occurred (CTC °III) – this patient had been heavily pretreated, and the cause of this polyneuropathy remains still unclear. No mucositis except for a light flush of the mucosa occurred, and all patients were able to eat at all times.

Chimerism, as analysed by short tandem repeat determination or FISH XY, reached more than 95% donor chimerism in all patients, except two, by d +14 and > 97% by d +28. One of these patients had a therapy-refractory CLL (lymphocyte counts, however, are decreasing continuously after transplantation), and one patient in a second chronic phase of a CML had a primary graft failure. He recovered with his own haematopoiesis by day +4. Once complete chimerism was reached, it was stable in all patients analysed so far, with two exceptions, both in patients with CML. One patient, while still on immunosuppression, could be reverted back to a complete cytogenetic and molecular remission and full donor chimerism by discontinuation of immunosuppression. The other patient required repeated donor lymphocyte infusions (DLI), and only after the addition of interferon and GM-CSF after DLI was a complete cytogenetic and molecular remission as well as complete donor chimerism reached again.

Acute GvHD exceeding °II was observed in 2 patients (1 MRD III° and 1 misMRD IV°) only. Twelve of 23 patients remained without signs of aGvHD. Limited cGvHD was observed in 3 and extensive cGvHD in 4 out of 16 patients.

Five out of 25 patients have died after transplantation. Four patients died of virus infections or apoplectic stroke (1) by day +28, day +111, day +202 and day +235 respectively. Three of them had a misMRD or MUD. One patient with a multiple myeloma and a severe cardiac amyloidosis suffered a cardiac arrest by day +61.

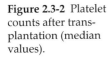

Figure 2.3-2 Platelet counts after transplantation (median values).

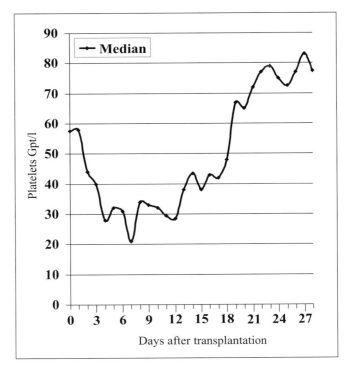

Conclusions

Summing up, the conditioning regimen with treosulfan and fludarabine was very well tolerated, especially taking into account the risk features of the patients, such as age, concurrent diseases (e.g. cardiac amyloidosis), previous transplants and the donor status. Complete chimerism could be achieved in almost all patients, except for one patient with a therapy-refractory CLL (but showing decreasing leukocyte counts). Comparing the frequency of primary graft failures with other toxicity-reduced regimens, treosulfan and fludarabine seems to be quite effective and safe at the same time, since autologous recovery of the haematopoiesis occurred rapidly in each patient involved [5].

Considering the low relapse rate (2/25 patients) and the risk status of the patients, the anti-leukaemic activity of treosulfan and fludarabine seems to be rather well developed. Relapsing patients were cured by the GvL effect either by withdrawal of the immunosuppression or by DLI. Other aims of a modern, conditioning regimen were achieved as well: fast haematologic recovery with low infection rate during neutropenia and no inappropriate degree of GvHD.

Presently, we feel that further careful evaluation of the treosulfan and fludarabine combination may lead to a promising toxicity-reduced conditioning regimen with sufficient stem cell toxicity, immunosuppression and anti-leukaemic activity.

References

1. BARRETT J., CHILDS R.: Non-myeloablative stem cell transplants. Br J Haematol 111 (2000) 6–17.
2. GIRALT S., *et al.*: Non-myeloablative "mini transplants". Cancer Treat Res 101 (1999) 97–108.
3. GRIGG A., *et al.*: "Mini-allografts" for haematological malignancies: an alternative to conventional myeloablative marrow transplant. Aust N Z J Med 29 (1999) 308–314.
4. PLOEMACHER R.E., *et al.*: Treosulfan as an alternative conditioning agent in bone marrow transplantation. BMT 25 (2000) Suppl. 1 141 (Abstract).
5. SANDMAIER B.M., *et al.*: Nonmyeloablative transplants: preclinical and clinical results. Semin Oncol 27 (2000) 78–81.
6. SCHEULEN M.E., *et al.*: Clinical phase I dose escalation and pharmacokinetic study of high-dose chemotherapy with treosulfan and autologous peripheral blood stem cell transplantation in patients with advanced malignancies. Clin Cancer Res 6 (2000) 4209–4216.
7. SINGHAL S., *et al.*: Non-myeloablative allogeneic transplantation ("microallograft") for refractory myeloma after two preceding autografts: feasibility and efficacy in a patient with active aspergillosis. Bone Marrow Transplant 26 (2000) 1231–1233.

2.4 CMV Seropositivity of the Patient with or without Reactivation Is the Most Important Prognostic Factor for Survival and Treatment-Related Mortality in Stem Cell Transplantation from Unrelated Donors Using Pre-Transplant in vivo T-Cell Depletion with ATG

Kröger[1]*, N., T. Zabelina[1], W. Krüger[1], H. Renges[1], H. Stute[1], J. Schrum[1], H. Kabisch[1], C. Löliger[2], P. Schäfer[3], A. Hinke[4], A. R. Zander[1]

[1] Bone Marrow Transplantation and [2] Dept. of Transfusion Medicine and [3] Microbiology, University Hospital, Hamburg, Germany, 4 WISP Research Institute, Langenfeld, Germany.

* To whom correspondence should be addressed (nkroeger@uke.uni-hamburg.de)

Summary

We evaluated the serological status of cytomegalovirus (CMV) infection as a risk factor for survival and treatment-related mortality (TRM) in 125 patients allografted from unrelated donors between 1994 and 1999. In all patients pretransplant in vivo T-cell depletion was achieved using rabbit anti-thymocyte globulin (ATG). Only one patient had primary graft failure, and severe grade III/IV GvHD occurred in 14% of the patients. The overall survival (OS) at three years was 70% for CMV-negative patients (n = 76) and 29% in the seropositive cohort (n = 49) (p > 0.001). In a multivariate analysis CMV seropositivity remained an independent negative prognostic factor for OS (RR: 2.1; CI: 1.2–3.8; p = 0.014), besides age > 20 years (RR: 2.74; CI: 1.2–3.8; p = 0.004) and late leukocyte engraftment (RR: 2.4; CI: 1.2–4.9; p = 0.015). The TRM for all patients was 27%. Despite monitoring for CMV antigenaemia and despite pre-emptive therapy with ganciclovir in case of reactivation, seropositive patients had a three times higher risk of fatal, treatment-related complications than seronegative patients. In a multivariate analysis, CMV seropositivity remained the strongest independent negative factor for TRM (RR: 5.3; CI: 1.9–14.6; p = 0.002), followed by age > 20 years (RR: 4.8; CI: 1.3–18.1; p = 0.02) and delayed leukocyte engraftment (RR: 3.6; CI: 1.2–11; p = 0.02). The TRM was balanced in seropositive patients with (n = 27) or without (n = 22) CMV reactivation (44% vs. 50%). We conclude that CMV seropositivity, despite the pre-emptive ganciclovir therapy and even without reactivation, is a major negative prognostic factor with respect to survival as well as TRM in unrelated stem cell transplantation using pretransplant in vivo T-cell depletion with ATG.

Introduction

Bone marrow transplantation from unrelated donors is an accepted treatment for patients with a variety of haematologic malignancies, bone marrow failure syndromes, immunodeficiencies and metabolic disorders without HLA-identical siblings [1,3,15,22,31]. The international registry network includes more than 5 million HLA-typed volunteers, resulting in a probability of about 75% of finding at least HLA-A, -B, -DR matched donors. Unrelated bone marrow transplantation is, however, associated with a high incidence of acute and chronic graft-versus-host disease (GvHD), graft failure and infectious complications [21,24]. By matching recipients and donors by genomic typing for HLA class II antigens, the incidence of GvHD was improved compared to serological typing alone [27]. The use of T-cell depleted marrow in unrelated transplant has resulted in a lower incidence of severe GvHD but in a higher rate of graft failure [21]. *In vivo* T-cell depletion can be achieved by pretransplant therapy with anti-CD25 antibody or anti-thymocyte globulin [3,17,39]. We have recently shown that ATG as part of the preparative regimen in unrelated stem cell transplantation reduces the risk of severe acute and chronic GvHD and of graft failure without an obvious increase of relapse [23]. Factors known to influence the outcome of unrelated stem cell transplantation include HLA disparity [3,10,21,28,32], patient's age, disease status at transplantation [18,24], cell dose [18,34] and CMV seropositivity of the recipient [25,34,35]. Cytomegalovirus infection is a major cause of morbidity and mortality after allogeneic stem cell transplantation [35]. Since studies have shown that prophylactic antiviral therapy in seropositive patients or pre-emptive therapy based on positive antigenaemia reduces the incidence of severe CMV disease and might improve survival in CMV-positive patients, these approaches have become clinical practice [6,14,19,38].

We analysed factors – including the CMV status of donor and recipient – influencing OS, DFS, relapse and treatment-related mortality in 125 patients undergoing unrelated stem cell transplantation after pretransplant serotherapy with ATG.

Methods

Patients

For this study we recruited a cohort comprising 125 consecutive patients with unrelated donor stem cell grafts transplanted between March 1994 and December 1999 at the Eppendorf University Hospital in Hamburg. Written informed consent was received from each patient, and the study was approved by the local Ethics Committee. The patients' characteristics are shown in Table 2.4-1. The mean age of the recipients was 30 years (range 1–56). There were 74 males and 51 females. Median follow-up was 29 months (range 2–90).

AML in 1st CR, MDS (RA, RAS) as well as CML in 1st chronic phase and haemophagocytic lymphohistiocytosis were considered to be standard risk, whereas MDS (RAEB, RAEB-T), AML beyond 1st CR, CML beyond 1st chronic phase and ALL beyond 1st CR or Philadelphia chromosome positivity were classified as high-risk disease.

HLA-A and -B antigens where typed by serologic methods and HLA-DRB1 alleles with sequence-specific oligonucleotide probes. Donors were required to match the recipients for the serologically defined HLA-A and -B antigens as well

Table 2.4-1 Characteristics of 125 patients.

Number of patients		125
Mean age of patients		33 (1-56)
Gender (male / female)		74 / 51
Median follow-up		29 months (1-91)
Diagnosis	Chronic myelogenous leukaemia	54
	• 1st chronic phase	48
	• 2nd chronic phase	1
	• accelerated phase	4
	• in blastic crisis	1
	Acute myeloid leukaemia	19
	• 1st CR	5
	• > 1st CR	14
	Myeloid dysplasia	8
	Acute lymphoblastic leukaemia (high-risk, Philadelphia-positive)	26
	• 1st CR	11
	• > 1st CR	15
	Biphenotypic acute leukaemia	1
	Multiple Myeloma	1
	Juvenile myelomonocytic leukaemia	2
	Malignant lymphoma in progress	1
	Familiar lymphocytic haemophagocytosis	9
	Inherited storage disease	4
CMV status patient / donor	Seronegative / seronegative	55
	Seronegative / seropositive	21
	Seropositive / seronegative	33
	Seropositive / seropositive	16
Conditioning	TBI – Cy	26
	TBI – Cy – VP	34
	Bu – Cy	34
	Bu – Cy – VP	23
	TMI – Bu (12 mg/kg) – Cy	1
	Other	7
HLA-Typing	Identical	107
	HLA-A mismatch	2
	HLA-B mismatch	7
	HLA-DRB1 mismatch	7
	Two mismatches	2
Cell source	BMT	107
	PBSCT	18
Transplanted cells (median)	MNC (x 10^8 / kg)	1.6 (0.4-51)
	CD34+ (x 10^6 / kg)	4.5 (0.6-30)

as HLA-DRB1 alleles. There were 107 patients with complete match for HLA-A, -B and -DRB1; 18 patients were mismatched in either HLA-B or HLA-DRB1 (Table 2.4-1).

Transplant-preparative regimen and GvHD prophylaxis

Twenty-six patients were conditioned with total-body irradiation, 1200 cGy given over three days in six fractions, followed by cyclophosphamide

(120 mg/kg), and 34 patients received TBI and cyclophosphamide plus etoposide (30–45 mg/kg). Thirty-four patients received busulfan (16 mg/kg) and cyclo-phosphamide (120 mg/kg). Twenty-three patients received busulfan (16 mg/kg), cyclophosphamide (120 mg/kg) and etoposide (30–45 mg/kg). Five patients received busulfan, cyclophosphamide and melphalan. Single patients received busulfan (16 mg/kg) plus etoposide (30 mg/kg), or total marrow irradiation (9 Gy), busulfan (12 mg/kg) and cyclophosphamide (120 mg/kg), or total-body irradiation plus etoposide. The stem cell source was bone marrow in 107 patients and peripheral blood stem cells in 18 patients. No manipulation of the graft was performed.

The GvHD prophylaxis consisted of cyclosporine A (3 mg/kg, given from day –1 to six months post transplantation). The dose of cyclosporine A was adjusted to cyclosporine A serum levels of 200–300 ng/ml. Cyclosporine A was tapered from day 84 and discontinued at day 180. Methotrexate (10 mg/m^2) was given at day 1, 3 and 6 post transplantation. Rabbit anti-human thymocyte-globulin (Fresenius, Bad Homburg, Germany) was given in 104 patients at a dose of 30 mg/kg over 12 hours on day –3, –2 and –1, and in 21 patients at a cumulative dose of ATG between 20 and 60 mg/kg. One patient received a cumulative ATG dose of 120 mg/kg. All patients received intravenous globulin (on day 1, 7, 14, 21, 28, 56, 84 and day 120). Ninety-one patients received IgM-enriched immunoglobulin (Pentaglobin) (Biotest, Frankfurt, Germany) and 34 patients immunoglobulin without IgM enrichment (Octagam, Octapharm, Dessau, Germany) on day 1, 7, 14, 21 and 28. 120 patients received, in addition, metronidazole (Clont, Bayer, Leverkusen, Germany) at a dose of 400 mg i.v., given 3 times a day, from conditioning until discharge. Standard criteria were used for acute and chronic GvHD [30]. Acute GvHD was treated with high-dose steroid, and extensive chronic GvHD with cyclosporine A and steroids. Chronic GvHD was evaluated in patients who survived at least 80 days with sustained engraftment.

Supportive care

All patients were nursed in single rooms with HEPA-filtered air. Antibiotic prophylaxis consisted of ofloxacin or ciprofloxacin, and antifungal prophylaxis of fluconazole, and – in case of prior mycotic infection – of amphotericin. Aciclovir was given as herpes prophylaxis from day 1 until day 180. Pneumo-cystis-carinii prophylaxis consisted of either trimethoprim/sulfamethoxazole or monthly inhalation with pentamidine.

All red blood products were irradiated before infusion, and patients with seronegativity for CMV received only blood products from CMV-negative donors.

Weekly monitoring of peripheral blood leukocytes (PBL) and urine by polymerase chain reaction (PCR) and CMV-shell vial culture was carried out. In addition, PBL were analysed weekly with a CMV pp65 antigenaemia assay. In case of positivity, ganciclovir treatment was initiated (5 mg/kg bw, IV, twice daily), and discontinued after negative test results were obtained. Patients with a high number of positive cells usually received 14 days maintenance therapy with 5 mg/kg ganciclovir, once daily. Patients with persistence of CMV antigenaemia were treated with foscarnet (2×60 mg/kg, daily) or a combination of ganciclovir (5 mg/kg) and foscarnet (90 mg/kg), daily. Patients with CMV disease additionally received CMV hyperimmunoglobulin. CMV disease was defined as pneumonia with positive CMV testing in BAL, or enteritis/hepatitis with positive histology (performed with *in situ* hybridization). All patients with pneumonia underwent bronchoscopy, and patients with enteritis, coloscopy. Patients with unclear hepatitis were subjected to percutaneous or transjugular liver biopsy.

All patients received haematopoietic growth factors (G-CSF, 5 μg/kg) intravenously beginning on day 1 and continued until the absolute granulocyte count was > 1.0/nl for three consecutive days. Prostaglandin E1 (Prostavasine, Schwarz-Pharma, Mannheim, Germany) at a dose of $500\,\mu$g was given daily as continuous infusion for patients with VOD hepatotoxicity upon a rise of total bilirubine above 2.0 mg/dL.

CMV-PCR

The polymerase chain reaction was performed as described by EINSELE et al. [11].

Shell vial culture

Quantitative virus culture was performed essentially as described [36]. Briefly, MRC-5 cell monolayers grown in shell vials were inoculated with 10^6 leukocytes or $200\,\mu$l of sterile-filtered urine by centrifugation at $700 \times g$ for 45 minutes. After incubation at 37 °C for 48 h cells were paraformaldehyde-fixed and permeabilized. Infected fibroblasts were visualized by indirect immuno-fluorescence staining using a monoclonal antibody (9221, DuPont de Nemours, Bad Homburg, Germany) directed against the CMV immediate early antigen p72.

Pp65 antigenaemia

Ten millilitres of whole blood were collected in EDTA tubes. Peripheral blood leukocytes were isolated as described previously [33] and quantitated with a haematological cell counter. Aliquots of 10^5 leukocytes each were centrifuged onto duplicate glass slides, paraformaldehyde-fixed and permeabilized, and pp65 antigens were detected in leukocytes by indirect immunofluorescence as described previously [13] using Clonab CMV monoclonal antibody (Biotest, Dreieich, Germany) following the manufacturers' instructions. Results were expressed as the total number of pp65-positive cells in 2×10^5 leukocytes.

Statistical methods

Disease-free survival, relapse-free survival and overall survival were calculated from start of therapy to the respective event. Death of whatever cause was counted as an event in case of disease-free survival, contrary to relapse-free survival with censoring of all deaths not caused by the underlying disease. All time-to-event curves were estimated according to the method of Kaplan and Meier and compared univariately using the log-rank test [29]. The chi-square test was used for univariate analysis of treatment-related mortality. Multivariate analyses of mortality-rate and event-type data were performed with the logistic and proportional hazard model respectively [9]. For correlation analysis, the Spearman-rank test was calculated. A p-value of < 0.05 was considered to be significant.

Results

Engraftment and graft failure

Only 1 patient with CML and blast crisis had a primary graft failure, and was unsuccessfully retransplanted on day 51 after the first transplantation, from the same donor; 6 patients died of treatment-related mortality before engraftment. The median number of marrow mononuclear cells given was 1.6×10^8 per kg (range 0.4–50.0). The median number of transplanted $CD34^+$ cells was 4.5×10^6 per kg (range 0.6–30.7). The median time to reach the leukocyte count $1.0 \times 10^9/l$ was 16 days (range 11–45). Eighty-six patients were evaluable for platelet engraftment: Platelet count $> 20 \times 10^9/l$ with platelet transfusion independence was reached at a median of 25 days (range 13–121). The number of infused $CD34^+$ cells ($r = 0.2$, $p = 001$) and MNCs ($r = 0.2$, $p = 0.004$) correlated with leukocyte engraftment as well as with platelet engraftment ($r = 0.2$, $p = 0.001$, and $r = 0.3$, $p = 0.004$, respectively).

GvHD

Sixteen patients had grade I acute GvHD, and grade II–IV acute GvHD occurred in 43 patients (34%). Severe grade III and IV GvHD developed in 18 patients (14%), 7 of whom died of acute GvHD. Chronic GvHD was evaluated in 91 patients who survived day 80 post BMT. The incidence of chronic GvHD was only 33%, 14 patients had limited disease (15%), and only 16 patients had extensive GvHD (18%) and required further immunosuppression consisting of prednisone or cyclosporine A.

Cytomegalovirus-serostatus and infection

Fifty-five patients (44%) were seronegative with a seronegative donor (R–/D–), whereas 21 patients (17%) were seronegative with a seropositive donor (R–/D+). The combination recipient positive/donor positive (R+/D+) was seen in 16 (13%) and recipient positive/donor negative (R+/D–) in 33 cases (26%). Overall, 27 patients (22%) developed CMV reactivation with positive PCR and/or a positive pp65-test. Six patients died of CMV pneumonitis. If the recipient was CMV-positive prior to transplantation, the probability of CMV reactivation was 55%, whereas no infection was seen in the combination R–/D–, and only 1 case of reactivation (5%) was seen after transplantation in R–/D+ constellation (Table 2.4-2).

Table 2.4-2 CMV serostatus of recipient/donor and CMV reactivity after transplantation.

CMV Serostatus	Recipient positive/ Donor positive	Recipient positive/ Donor negative	Recipient negative/ Donor positive	Recipient negative/ Donor negative
Number	16	33	21	55
CMV reactivation	6 (38%)	21 (61%)	1 (5%)	0

Overall survival

After a median follow-up of 29 months (range 2–90), the estimated overall survival at three years for all patients is 57% (CI 95%: 47–67%). The Kaplan-Meier survival curves for overall and disease-free survival are shown in Figures 2.4-1, 2.4-2 and 2.4-3.

In a univariate analysis, overall survival was significantly better for patients with CMV seronegativity (p = 0.00009), low-risk disease status at transplantation (p = 0.001), rapid leukocyte engraftment within 20 days after transplantation (p = 0.004) and age < 20 years (p = 0.02). No significant difference in overall survival was found between HLA-matched and HLA-mismatched transplantation, for infused CD34+ cells/kg (above or below 3×10^6/kg) or MNCs, gender and age of the donor, sex-match between recipient and donor, dose of ATG, incidence of acute and chronic GvHD (Table 2.4-3). According to multivariate analysis, the factors for impaired overall survival which remained significant were CMV seropositivity of the recipient (RR: 2.1; CI: 1.2–3.8; p = 0.014), patient age > 20 years (RR: 2.7; CI: 1.2–3.8; p = 0.004), leukocyte engraftment beyond 20 days after transplantation (RR: 2.4; CI: 1.2–4.9; p = 0.015), and high-risk disease status (RR: 3.4; CI : 1.8–4.9; p = 0.0001) (Table 2.4-4).

Disease-free survival

The estimated disease-free survival at three years is 49% (CI 95%: 39–59%). In a univariate analysis disease-free survival was significantly better for patients with CMV seronegativity (p = 0.0001), low risk disease status at transplantation (p = 0.003), rapid leukocyte engraftment within 20 days after transplantation

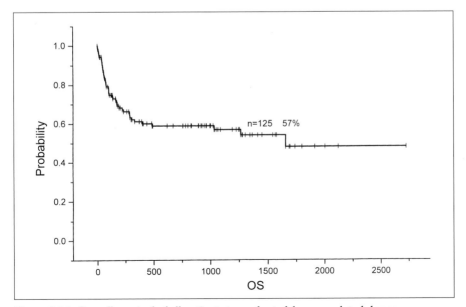

Figure 2.4-1 Overall survival of all patients transplanted from unrelated donor.

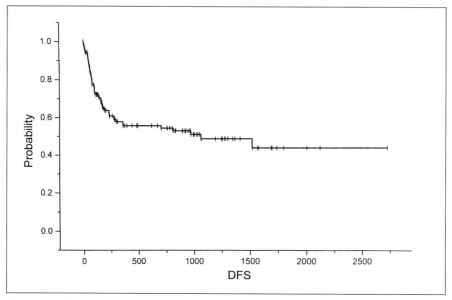

Figure 2.4-2 Disease-free survival (DFS) of all patients transplanted from unrelated donor.

Table 2.4-3 Univariate analysis of overall survival, disease-free survival and treatment-related mortality and relapse.

		OS	DFS	TRM	Relapse
HLA-matched vs. mismatched		n.s.	n.s.	n.s.	n.s.
CD34+ cells:	< 3 x 10⁶/kg vs.> 3 x 10⁶/kg	n.s.	n.s.	n.s.	n.s.
PBSC vs. BM		n.s.	n.s	n.s.	n.s.
Gender donor:	female vs. male	n.s.	n.s.	n.s.	n.s.
Age donor:	< 30 years > 30 years	n.s.	n.s.	n.s.	n.s.
ATG	< 90 mg/kg vs. 90 mg/kg	n.s.	n.s.	n.s.	n.s.
Leukocyte 1/μl	< 20 days vs.> 20 days	0.004	0.007	0.007	n.s.
Platelet 20/μl:	< 25 days vs.> 25 days	n.s.	n.s.	n.s.	n.s.
Acute GvHD vs. non-aGvHD		n.s.	n.s.	n.s.	n.s.
Chronic GvHD vs. non-cGvHD		n.s.	n.s.	n.s.	n.s.
Recipient CMV+ vs. CMV–		< 0.0001	0.0001	< 0.0001	
Donor CMV+ vs. CMV–		n.s.	n.s.	n.s.	n.s.
Disease stage: high-risk vs. low-risk		0.001	0.003	n.s.	0.003
Recipient age:	< 20 years vs.> 20 years	0.02	0.02	0.002	n.s.

(p = 0.007) and age < 20 years (p = 0.02). No difference in disease-free survival was observed for HLA-matched/-mismatched transplantation, for infused CD34+ cells/kg (above or below 3 x 10⁶/kg) or MNCs, gender and age of the donor, sex-match between recipient and donor, dose of ATG, incidence of acute and chronic GvHD. According to multivariate analysis, the factors for disease-free survival were CMV seropositivity of the recipient (RR: 2.0; CI: 1.2–3.6; p = 0.013), patient age < 20 years (RR: 2.6; CI: 1.4–5.0; p = 0.004), high-risk disease

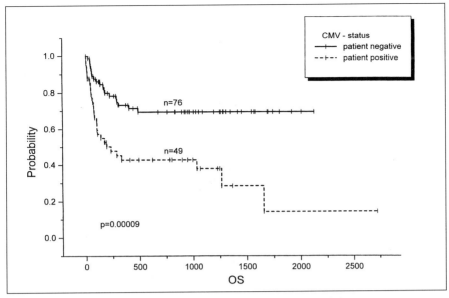

Figure 2.4-3 Overall survival (OS) related to the CMV serostatus of the recipient.

Table 2.4-4 Multivariate analysis of unfavourable factors for OS, DFS, and relapse.

	Overall survival			Disease-free survival			Relapse		
	RR	95% CI	p-value	RR	95% CI	p-value	RR	95% CI	p-value
Recipient CMV positivity	2.11	1.16-3.84	0.014	2.04	1.17-3.57	0.013	1.22	0.49-3.02	n.s.
Recipient age: > 20 years	2.74	1.16-3.84	0.004	2.59	1.36-4.94	0.004	1.85	0.72-4.75	n.s.
Disease stage: high-risk	3.40	1.79-6.47	0.0001	3.00	1.65-5.43	0.0003	3.73	1.40-9.95	0.008
Leukocyte* > 1/µl > 20 days	2.40	1.18-4.87	0.015	2.21	1.09-4.15	0.027	1.43	0.51-4.04	n.s.

* based on 116 patients

status (RR: 3.0; CI: 1.7–5.4; p = 0.0003) and leukocyte engraftment < 20 days after transplantation (RR: 2.2; CI: 1.1–4.2; p = 0.027) (Tables 2.4-3 and 2.4-4).

Relapse

After a median follow-up of 29 months 21 relapses were observed (17%). Relapse occurred after a median of 8 months (range 2–51) post transplantation. The only risk factor which was significant for relapse in a multivariate analysis was high-risk disease status at transplantation (RR: 3.7; CI: 1.4–10.0; p = 0.008) (Table 2.4-4).

Treatment-related mortality

There were 34 deaths (27%) due to treatment. The principal causes of death are summarized in Table 2.4-6. Infection was the major cause of death occurring in

Table 2.4-5 Multivariate analysis of unfavourable factors for treatment-related mortality.

Variables	RR	95% CI	p-value
Recipient CMV-positivity	5.25	1.89-14.60	0.002
Leukocyte* > $1/\mu l$ > 20 days	3.66	1.21-11.04	0.024
Donor CMV-positivity	0.55	0.09-3.28	n.s.
Recipient age > 20 years	4.82	1.29-18.07	0.022

* = based on 116 patients

18 patients: Fungal infections (n = 10), viral (cytomegalovirus) infections (n = 6) or bacterial sepsis (n = 3). One fatal EBV-related lymphoma was observed. The remaining patients died of GvHD (n = 7) or toxicity, especially VOD, bleeding or interstitial pneumonia (n = 8). In univariate analyses, CMV seropositivity of the recipient (p < 0.0001), age > 20 years (p = 0.0024), and leukocyte engraftment later than 20 days (p = 0.007) were significant risk factors for treatment-related mortality. No significance was noted for transplanted CD34+ cell dose, CMV seropositivity of the donor, disease risk status prior to transplantation, gender mismatch, gender of the donor, HLA mismatch, source of stem cell, incidence of acute and chronic GvHD, and dose of ATG. According to multivariate analysis, the only factors of interest for increased treatment-related mortality remained CMV seropositivity of the recipient (RR: 5.3; CI: 1.9–14.6; p = 0.002), age > 20 years (RR: 4.8; CI: 1.3–18.1; p = 0.02) and leukocyte engraftment > 20 days (RR: 3.6; CI: 1.2–11.0; p = 0.02) (Table 2.4-5). The treatment-related mortality in CMV-seronegative patients was 14% and in seropositive patients 47%. In seropositive patients with reactivation (n = 27, pp65- or PCR-positive), the main cause of death was due to CMV disease, especially pneumonitis in 5 cases, followed by GvHD (n = 3), fungal infection (n = 1), sepsis (n = 1) and EBV-related lymphoma (n = 1), resulting in a TRM-rate of 44%. However, patients with CMV seropositivity without reactivation (n = 22) also had a high mortality (50%), which was mainly due to toxicity (n = 4) and infections (n = 6) (Table 2.4-6). After the censoring of 5 patients who died before day 30 the treatment-related mortality rate was still 28% in this subgroup. Five out of 6 CMV-seropositive patients who developed fatal CMV pneumonitis despite pre-emptive ganciclovir therapy were transplanted by a CMV-negative donor. In a univariate analysis of the CMV-seropositive subgroup, age > 20 years was the sole risk factor for treatment-related mortality (p = 0.03), whereas incidence of GvHD, HLA mismatch, transplanted CD34+ cell-dose or stem cell source could not be identified as a risk factor for TRM.

Discussion

In this study of unrelated stem cell transplantation with anti-thymocyte globulin administered prior to transplantation for *in vivo* T-cell depletion, we confirm the observation that CMV seropositivity of the recipient is a major adverse risk factor in unrelated stem cell transplantation with respect to overall and disease-free survival as well as to treatment-related mortality [25,35]. For overall and disease-free survival CMV positivity had the strongest negative predictive

Table 2.4-6 Causes of treatment-related mortality with respect to different CMV serostatus of the donor.

	CMV-negative	CMV-positive with reactivation	CMV-positive without reactivation
	n = 6	n = 27	n = 22
GvHD	3	3	1
Fungal infection	5	1	4
VOD	1	-	2
CMV-disease	-	6	-
Graft failure	1	-	-
EBV-Lymphoma	-	1	-
Alveolar haemorrhage	1	-	1
Bleeding	-	-	1
Sepsis	-	1	2
Median days from transplantation	65 (21–171)	112 (50–231)	64 (2–99)
Overall	11 (14.5%)	12 (44%)	11 (50%)

value, followed by age, late engraftment (> 20 days) and disease risk status at transplantation. CMV positivity strongly predicted for TRM, followed by age and leukocyte engraftment.

CMV infection and CMV-related disease are major complications after allogeneic stem cell transplantation with a high mortality rate, especially in case of interstitial pneumonia [12,26]. The known risk factors for CMV reactivity and disease are CMV seropositivity of the recipient/donor, acute GvHD, HLA mismatch, age and T-cell depletion [2,7,12,26,37]. In our study 55% of the CMV-seropositive patients developed CMV reactivation requiring pre-emptive ganciclovir therapy, which is in accordance with the previously published results [2,19,26,37]. However, only 1 out of 21 seronegative recipients with seropositive donor experienced CMV reactivation (5%), which is in contrast to 57% reported earlier from the Seattle group. This low incidence of reactivation might also be due to the use of CMV-seronegative blood products and filtering of leukocytes, which has reduced the transmission of CMV by transfusion[14]. Within the group of CMV-seropositive recipients, those with seropositive donors had a better overall survival than those with seronegative donors (37% vs. 28%) and a lower frequency of CMV reactivation by pp65-positive antigenaemia (38% vs. 61%). Furthermore, it is noteworthy that 5 out of 6 seropositive patients who died of CMV pneumonia had a seronegative donor. Therefore, in unrelated stem cell transplantation for seropositive recipients, a seropositive donor seems to be more appropriate than a seronegative one. This is in accordance with the observation of BOLAND *et al.*, who reported in CMV-seropositive patients with a seropositive donor an earlier lymphocyte proliferative response to CMV than in CMV-positive recipients with a seronegative marrow donor [6]. Treatment-related mortality in CMV-seropositive recipients was 47% in comparison to 15% in the CMV-seronegative group, which compares with the recently reported TRM in allogeneic, partially

T-cell depleted stem cell transplantation [7]. This group reported a treatment-related mortality rate of 18% for the CMV-negative and 42% for CMV-positive patients. In several studies, ganciclovir, as prophylaxis or as pre-emptive therapy, is able to reduce CMV disease and CMV disease-related mortality [5,11,16,38]. However, in randomized trials, when comparing prophylactic ganciclovir therapy with placebo in CMV-positive patients, the day 100 mortality was balanced in both groups, despite a reduction of CMV reactivation and CMV disease in the ganciclovir arm [16,38]. In our study, the CMV positivity of the recipient was the strongest factor for increased TRM, despite pre-emptive ganciclovir therapy in pp65-positive patients. The negative impact of CMV positivity on TRM, despite pre-emptive therapy, has been recently reported in allogeneic, related stem cell transplantation [7], showing, however, a strong association with the incidence of acute GvHD. In our study of unrelated transplantation, acute GvHD had no influence on overall and disease-free survival, nor on TRM; and CMV positivity was not a risk factor for developing aGvHD. Another, even more important finding is that the mortality rate of CMV-positive patients is as high in cases without reactivation as it is with reactivation, suggesting that CMV positivity is, in itself, an independent risk factor for TRM. What are the factors influencing the higher TRM in CMV-positive patients, if CMV disease can be prevented by pre-emptive therapy or in patients without any sign of reactivation (negative PCR or pp65 antigenaemia)? While the mortality of CMV-positive patients with reactivation is due mainly to CMV-related diseases, and occurs after a median of 112 days post transplantation, the high mortality rate of CMV-positive patients without reactivation was due mainly to toxicity like VOD, sepsis, bleeding, alveolar haemorrhage or fungal infection, and occurred earlier in the post-transplant period (median 64 days). In a subanalysis of CMV-positive patients for risk factors for TRM only age > 20 years was a risk factor in univariate analysis with borderline significance (p = 0.03), while no influence was seen for factors like GvHD, HLA mismatch, transplanted CD34$^+$ cell dose or stem cell source. The relatively low numbers of included patients should, however, be kept in mind.

We conclude that CMV seropositivity, despite pre-emptive ganciclovir therapy, or even without reactivation, has a major negative prognostic impact for overall and disease-free survival, as well as for TRM in unrelated stem cell transplantation using pretransplant *in vivo* T-cell depletion with ATG. Furthermore, the strongest factor for TRM remains CMV positivity of the patient with or without reactivation. In unrelated stem cell transplantation with *in vivo* T-cell depletion, a seropositive donor should be preferred to a seronegative one when confronted with CMV-seropositive patients. Sustaining the efforts needed to prevent CMV infection and CMV disease, further investigations are justified considering the high mortality suffered by CMV-seropositive patients facing unrelated stem cell transplantation.

Acknowledgements

We thank the staff of the BMT unit for providing excellent care for our patients, and the medical technicians for their brilliant work in the BMT laboratory.

References

1. ANASETTI , C., *et al.*: Effect of HLA incompatibility on graft versus host disease, relapse, and survival after marrow transplantation for patients with leukemia and lymphoma. Hum Immunol 29 (1990) 79–84.

2. BACIGALUPO, A., *et al.*: CMV antigenemia after allogeneic bone marrow transplantation: correlation of CMV-antigen positive cell number with transplant-related mortality. Bone Marrow Transplant 16 (1995) 155–161.

3. BAURMANN, H., *et al.*: Potent effect of ATG as part of the conditioning in matched unrelated donor (MUD) transplantation. Blood 92 (Suppl 1) (1998) 290a.

4. BEATTY, P.G., *et al.*: Marrow transplantation from related donors other than HLA-identical siblings. N Engl J Med 313 (1985) 765–771.

5. BOECKH, H., *et al.*: Cytomegalovirus pp65 antigenemia-guided early treatment with ganciclovir versus ganciclovir at engraftment after allogeneic marrow transplantation. Blood 88 (1996) 4063–4070.

6. BOLAND, G.N., *et al.*: Evidence of transfer of cellular and humoral immunity to cytomegalovirus from donor to recipient in allogeneic bone marrow transplantation. Clin Exp Immunol 88 (1992) 506–512.

7. BROERS, A.E.C., *et al.*: Increased transplant-related morbidity and mortality in CMV seropositive patients despite highly effective prevention of CMV disease after allogeneic T-cell depleted stem cell transplantation. Blood 95 (2000) 2240–2245.

8. COURIEL, D., *et al.*: Early reactivation of cytomegalovirus and high risk of interstitial pneumonia following T-cell depleted BMT for adults with heamatological malignancies. Bone Marrow Transplant 18 (1996) 347–351.

9. COX, D.R.: Regression models and life tables. J Roy Stat Soc (B) 34 (1972) 187–202.

10. DAVIES, S., *et al.*: Unrelated donor bone marrow transplantation: influence of HLA-A and B incompatibility on outcome. Blood 6 (1995) 1636–1642.

11. EINSELE, H., *et al.*: Polymerase chain reaction monitoring reduces the incidence of cytomegalovirus disease and the duration of side effects of antiviral therapy after bone marrow transplantation. Blood 86 (1995) 2815–2821.

12. FORMAN, S.J., ZAIA, J.A. Treatment and prevention of cytomegalovirus pneumonia after bone marrow transplantation: Where do we stand? Blood 83 (1994) 2392–2398.

13. GERNA, G., *et al.*: Comparison of different immunostaining techniques and monoclonal antibodies to the lower matrix phosphoprotein (pp65) for optimal quantitation of human cytomegalovirus antigenaemia. J Clin Microbiol 30 (1992) 1232–1237.

14. GILBERT, G.L., *et al.*: Prevention of transfusion-acquired cytomegalovirus infection in infants by blood filtration to remove leukocytes. Lancet 1 (1989) 1228–1233.

15. GOLDMAN, J.M., *et al.*: Bone marrow transplantation for chronic myelogenous leukemia in chronic phase: increased risk of relapse associated with T-cell depletion. Ann Intern Med 108 (1988) 806–814.

16. GOODRICH, J.M., *et al.*: Ganciclovir prophylaxis to prevent cytomegalovirus disease after allogeneic marrow transplant. Ann Intern Med 118 (1993) 173–178.

17. HALE, G., *et al.*: Improving the outcome of bone marrow transplantation by using CD52 monoclonal antibodies to prevent graft versus host disease and graft rejection. Blood 92 (1998) 4581–4590.

18. HANSEN, J.A., *et al.*: Bone marrow transplants from unrelated donors for patients with chronic myeloid leukemia. N Engl J Med 338 (1998) 962–968.

19. HERTENSTEIN, B., *et al.*: In vivo/ex vivo T cell depletion of GvHD prophylaxis influences onset and course of active cytomegalovirus infection and disease after BMT. Bone Marrow Transplant 15 (1995) 387–393.

20. KAPLAN, E.L., MEIER, P.: Nonparametric estimation from incomplete observations. J Am Stat Ass 53: (1958) 457–460.

21. KERNAN, N.A., *et al.*: Analysis of 462 transplantations from unrelated donors facilitated by the national marrow donor program. N Engl J Med 328 (1993) 593–602.

22. KRIVIT, W., *et al.*: State of art review. Bone marrow transplantation treatment for storage diseases. Bone Marrow Transplant (Suppl 1) 10 (1992) 87–92.

23. KRÖGER, N., *et al.*: Anti-Thymocyte-Globulin as part of the preparative regimen prevents acute and chronic Graft versus Host disease (GvHD) in allogeneic stem cell transplantation from unrelated donors. Ann Haematol (2001) (in press).

24. McGLAVE, P., *et al.*: Unrelated donor marrow transplantation for chronic myelogenous leukemia: Initial experience of the National Marrow Donor Program. Blood 81 (1993) 543–550.

25. McGLAVE, P.B., *et al.*: Unrelated donor marrow transplantation for chronic myelogenous leukemia: 9 years experience of the National Marrow Donor Program. Blood 95 (2000) 2219–2225.

26. MEYERS. J.D., *et al.*: Risk factors for cytomegalovirus infection after human marrow transplantation. J Infect Dis 153 (1989) 478–488.

27. NADEMANEE, A., *et al.*: The outcome of matched unrelated donor bone marrow transplantation in patients with heamatologic malignancies using molecular typing for donor selection and graft versus host disease prophylaxis regimen of ciclosporine, methotrexate, and prednisone. Blood 86 (1995) 1228–1234.

28. PETERSDORF, E., *et al.*: The significance of HLA-DRB1 matching on clinical outcome after HLA-A, B, DR identical unrelated donor marrow transplantation. Blood 86 (1995) 1606–1613.

29. PETO, R., PETO, J.: Asymptomatically efficient rank invariation test procedures. J R Stat Soc A 135: (1972) 185–206.

30. PRZEPIORKA, K.M., *et al.*: 1994 Consensus Conference on acute GvHD-grading. Bone Marrow Transplant 15 (1995) 825–831.

31. RAMSAY, N.K.C., DAVIES, S.: Bone marrow transplantation for acute leukemia. Baillieres Clinical Haematol 4 (1991) 483–491.

32. SAZASUKI, T., *et al.*: Effect of matching class I alleles on clinical outcome after transplantation of heamatopoietic cells from unrelated donor. N Engl J Med 399 (1998) 1177–1181.

33. SCHÄFER, P., *et al.*: Minimal effect of delayed sample processing on results of quantitative PCR for cytomegalovirus DNA in leucocytes compared to results of an antigenaemia assay. J Clin Microbiol 35 (1997) 741–744.

34. SIERRA, J., *et al.*: Transplantation of marrow cells from unrelated donors for treatment of high-risk acute leukaemia. Effect of leukaemic burden, donor HLA-matching and marrow cell dose. Blood 89 (1997) 3590–3597.

35. SPENCER, A., *et al.*: Bone marrow transplantation for chronic myeloid leukemia with volunteer unrelated donors using ex vivo or in vivo T-cell depletion: major prognostic impact of HLA class I identity between donor and recipient. Blood 86 (1995) 3590–3597.

36. STORCH, G.A., *et al.*: Comparison of PCR and pp65 antigenaemia assay with quantitative shell vial culture for detection of cytomegalovirus in blood leucocytes from solid-organ transplant recipients. J Clin Microbiol 32 (1994) 997–1003.

37. TRENSCHEL, R., *et al.*: Reduced risk of persisting cytomegalovirus pp65 antigenemia and cytomegalovirus interstitial pneumonia following allogeneic PBST. Bone Marrow Transplant 25 (2000) 665–672.

38. WINSTON, D.J., *et al.*: Ganciclovir prophylaxis of cytomegalovirus infection and disease in allogeneic bone marrow transplant recipients. Ann Intern Med 118 (1993) 179.

39. ZANDER, A.R., *et al.*: Use of a five-agent GvHD prevention regimen in recipients of unrelated donor marrow. Bone Marrow Transplant 23 (1999) 889–893.

2.5 Total Body Irradiation versus Busulfan in Combination with Cyclophosphamide as Conditioning for Unrelated Stem Cell Transplantation in CML Patients. A Comparison

Zabelina[1], T., N. Kröger[1]*, W. Krüger[1], H. Renges[1], H. Kabisch[1], N. Jaburg[1], C. Löliger[2], A. Krüll[3], A. R. Zander[1]

[1] Bone Marrow Transplantation [2] Dept. of Transfusion Medicine, [3] Dept. of Radiation Therapy, Hamburg University Hospital, Germany

* To whom correspondence should be addressed (nkroeger@uke.uni-hamburg.de)

Summary

We compared fractionated total body irradiation (12 Gy)/cyclophosphamide (120 mg/kg) with busulfan (16 mg/kg)/cyclophosphamide (120 mg/kg) as preparative therapy in unrelated donor stem cell transplantation of CML patients.

Fifty patients with CML (1. CP = 46; aP = 4) and a median age of 36 years (range: 16–52) were enrolled in this sequential trial between 1994 and 1999. In both groups patients were well balanced with respect to age, disease status, stem cell source and CMV status. All patients received standard doses of cyclosporine A, methotrexate and anti-thymocyte globulin (ATG) as GvHD prophylaxis. No graft failures occurred in either group. The median day of leukocyte engraftment was earlier in the Bu/Cy than in the TBI/Cy group (day 15 vs. 17; $p = 0.006$). The incidence of grade II–IV GvHD was 40% in the TBI/Cy and 36% in the Bu/Cy group, whereas severe grade III/IV GvHD was only observed in 12% of patients in both groups. The incidence of chronic GvHD (limited and extensive) at 1 year was higher in the Bu/Cy arm (65% vs. 30%; $p = 0.02$). More toxicity grade I/II of the liver (88% vs. 44%; $p = 0.002$) and more haemorrhagic cystitis (32% vs. 8%; $p = 0.02$) were observed in the Bu/Cy regimen. Seven relapses in the TBI and no relapse in the Bu/Cy group were observed after a median follow-up of 44 and 15 months, respectively. The estimated 3-year OS and DFS was 72% (95% CI: 55–98%) and 58% (95% CI: 39–77%) in the TBI, and 70% (95% CI: 51–89%) for DFS and OS in the Bu/Cy group. We conclude that the anti-leukaemic effect of the Bu/Cy regimen seems to be at least as effective as the TBI/Cy combination in unrelated stem cell transplantation of CML patients, with no graft failures, but that it correlates with a higher incidence of liver toxicity, haemorrhagic cystitis and chronic GvHD. Longer follow-up is necessary to determine the late relapse rate and late toxicity.

Introduction

Allogeneic bone marrow transplantation is the only proven curative therapy for patients with chronic myeloid leukaemia. Only about 30% of candidates for allogeneic bone marrow transplantation have an HLA-identical sibling. Therefore, bone marrow transplantation from unrelated HLA-compatible donors has become an alternative option and is now considered as standard therapy for young patients with CML lacking a suitable sibling donor. However, the results of unrelated bone marrow transplantation compared to those from sibling donors seem to be inferior because of higher morbidity and mortality due to graft failure, infections and graft-versus-host disease (GvHD) [13,15]. Total body irradiation (TBI) in combination with cyclophosphamide is the most frequently used preparative regimen in unrelated bone marrow transplantation of CML [9,10,22]. The radiation-free regimen of busulfan and cyclophosphamide has been proven effective for eradication of leukaemia, and sufficiently immunosuppressive for engraftment in HLA-matched sibling transplantation. In randomized trials of Bu/Cy versus TBI/Cy in HLA-matched sibling trans-plantation of CML patients the combination of busulfan/cyclophosphamide was shown to be at least as effective as TBI/cyclophosphamide [5,6]. Furthermore, the French study [6] reported a higher antileukaemic effect and the Seattle group [5] a significantly lower toxicity of the busulfan/cyclophosphamide combination. In unrelated bone marrow transplantation, the TBI regimen is commonly used because TBI might be required to obtain the degree of immunosuppression needed for engraftment. In several single centre reports a 0% to 60% incidence of graft failure in unrelated bone marrow transplantation was observed using the busulfan/cyclophosphamide combination as preparation [4,11,16,23]. In the present study we report the results of 50 CML patients who underwent allogeneic unrelated stem cell transplantation between 1994 and 1999 at our centre. In this sequential trial patients transplanted before 1996 were treated with TBI/cyclophosphamide, whereas subsequent patients received busulfan/cyclophosphamide as conditioning.

Materials and methods

Patient population

The study group consisted of 50 patients with chronic myeloid leukaemia receiving unrelated donor stem cell transplants between 1994 and 1999 at the University Hospital Eppendorf in Hamburg. Written informed consent was obtained from each patient, and the study was approved by the local Ethics Committee. Both groups were well balanced with respect to age, CMV status, stem cell source and disease status. Patient characteristics are shown in Table 2.5-1.

HLA-typing and donor matching

HLA-A and -B antigens where typed by serological methods, HLA-DRB1 alleles were typed with sequence-specific oligonucleotide probes. In all patients, a pretransplantation lymphocyte cross-match with patient sera and donor cells was performed. There were 43 patients completely matched for HLA-B and -DRB1, and 7 patients were mismatched either at HLA-B or -DRB1.

Transplant preparative regimen

Twenty-five patients received conditioning with total-body irradiation, 1200 cGy given over three days in six fractions, and 25 patients received busulfan (14–16 mg/kg), both followed by cyclophosphamide (120 mg/kg). Busulfan was

Table 2.5-1 Patient Characteristics.

Variable	TBI/Cy (n = 25)	Bu/Cy (n = 25)	p-value
Median age (range)	36 (21-51)	36 (16-52)	n.s.
Median age of donor (range)	32 (19-50)	34 (23-57)	n.s.
Gender patients: m:f	14:11	15:10	n.s.
Gender donors: m:f	17:8	14:11	n.s.
BMT < 2 years from diagnosis	15	19	n.s.
BMT > 2 years from diagnosis	10	6	n.s.
Disease status:			n.s.
– 1. CP	22	24	
– Accelerated phase	3	1	
Sex donor/recipient: matched/mismatched	18:7	15:10	n.s.
HLA-matched	24	19	n.s.
– Mismatched:	1	6	0.04
– DRB1	1	3	
– HLA-B	0	3	
ABO:			
– identical	7	5	n.s.
– Non-identical	17	20	n.s.
Stem cell source:			
– BM	23	21	n.s.
– PBSC	2	4	n.s.
ATG dose: – 90 mg/kg	25	18	
– 60 mg/kg	–	1	
– 30 mg/kg	–	5	
– 20 mg/kg	–	1	
Median CD34+ cells x10^6/kg (range)	3.8 (0.6-17)*	3.7 (1.4- 10)**	n.s.
Median MNC x10^8/kg (range)	1.3 (0.4- 11)	1.3 (0.4- 14)	n.s.
CMV Status:			
– Positive (recipient and/or donor)	14	15	n.s.
– Negative (recipient and donor)	11	10	n.s.

* n = 20
** n = 24

administered orally in four divided doses daily for 4 days (day –8 to –5) and cyclophosphamide (60 mg/kg) was given intravenously over 1 hour for 2 days (day –4 and –3). Phenytoin was given to prevent busulfan-induced seizures for another 2 days after stopping busulfan. Uroepithelial prophylaxis was achieved with hyperhydration and mesna. Bone marrow or peripheral blood stem cells were infused on day 0. The stem cell source was bone marrow in 44 patients and peripheral blood stem cells in 6 patients. No manipulation of the graft was performed.

GvHD prophylaxis

GvHD prophylaxis using cyclosporine A was carried out as described in chapter 2.4, page 50. Anti-thymocyte globulin (rabbit, Fresenius, Bad Homburg, Germany) was given to all patients; 43 patients received a dose of 30 mg/kg over

12 hours on days –3, –2 and –1, and 7 patients received a cumulative dose of ATG ranging from 20 to 60 mg/kg. All patients received intravenous globulin on day 1, 3, 7, 14, 21, 28, 56, 84 and day 120. To prevent gut GvHD, metronidazole (Clont, Bayer, Leverkusen, Germany) at a dose of 500 mg i.v., was given 3 times a day from conditioning until discharge [25]. The standard criteria were used for grading acute and chronic GvHD [12]. Acute GvHD was treated with high-dose steroids, and extensive chronic GvHD with cyclosporine A and steroids. Chronic GvHD was evaluated in patients who survived at least 80 days with sustained engraftment.

Regimen-related toxicity

Regimen-related toxicity affecting the renal, hepatic, cardiac, pulmonary, gastrointestinal, CNS systems and mucous membranes was graded using the Bearman score [2]. The maximum score for each organ system was recorded. Attempts were made to exclude toxicities due to GvHD from therapy-related toxicity. Veno-occlusive disease of the liver was graded according to the Seattle criteria [14].

Supportive care

The procedure has been described in Chapter 2.4, page 50.

Statistical methods

Statistical analysis was performed by using WIN-STAT-software (Kalmia Co., Inc.; Cambridge, MA, USA). GvHD and survival were analysed by life table procedure according to the Kaplan-Meier method. Differences in survival and GvHD were studied using the log-rank test. For comparison, the independent t-test was used. A p-value of < 0.05 was considered significant.

Results

Engraftment

No graft failures were observed in either group. The median number of transplanted CD34$^+$ cells/kg was well balanced between the two groups: 3.8×10^6/kg in the TBI group and 3.7×10^6/kg in the Bu/Cy group (p = 0.4). However, leukocyte engraftment (> 1000/mm^3) was faster in the Bu/Cy group (median 15 [range: 11–20] versus 17 days [range: 12–24]) (p = 0.006). Platelet engraftment (> 20000/mm^3) was reached for Bu/Cy and for TBI/Cy after a median of 21 and 24 days, respectively (n. s., p = 0.2).

Graft-versus-host disease

Nine patients (36%) in the TBI/Cy group and 11 patients (44%) in the Bu/Cy group experienced no signs of acute GvHD. Thirteen patients (52%) in the TBI group and 11 (44%) patients in the Bu/Cy group developed mild acute GvHD grade I or II. Severe grade III/IV GvHD occurred in only 3 patients in each group (12%). Chronic GvHD was observed in 6 patients in the TBI/Cy and 11 patients in the Bu/Cy group, resulting in a probability of chronic GvHD at 1 year of 65% in the Bu/Cy and 30% in the TBI/Cy group (p = 0.02). Extensive chronic GvHD

Table 2.5-2 Results.

Variable	TBI/Cy (n = 25)	Bu/Cy (n = 25)	p-value
Acute GvHD:			
– Grade II–IV	40%	36%	n.s.
– Grade III/IV	12%	12%	n.s.
Chronic GvHD overall (at 1 year):	30%	65%	0.02
– Limited	17%	48%	n.s.
– Extensive	16%	33%	n.s.
Engraftment: median days (range):			
– Leukocyte > 1000/mm³	17 (12- 24)	15 (11- 20)	0.006
– Platelets > 20000/mm³	24 (15- 43)*	22 (13- 41)**	n.s.
Toxicity (Bearman):			
– Hepatic I/II	60%		0.002
– Renal I/II	35%		n.s.
– Mucositis II	96%		n.s.
Haemorrhagic cystitis	8%	32%	0.02
Veno-occlusive disease:		88%	
– Mild	1	44%	n.s.
– Moderate	8	96%	n.s.
TRM	20%	28%	n.s
3-years estimated OS	72%	70%	n.s.
3-years estimated DFS	58%	72%	n.s.

* n = 17
** n = 22
*** follow-up: TBI/Cy: 44 months and Bu/Cy: 15 months

was more common in the Bu/Cy arm (6 vs. 3 patients), even if patients with HLA-mismatched donors were censored.

Toxicity and treatment-related mortality

Toxicity of the liver grade I or II according to the Bearman scale was higher in the Bu/Cy than in the TBI group (88% vs. 44%; p = 0.002). Additionally, a trend for more moderate VOD was observed in the Bu/Cy group (56% vs. 32%; p = 0.1). Haemorrhagic cystitis was seen more often in the Bu/Cy arm (32% vs. 8%, p = 0.02). Other toxicities such as mucositis or renal toxicity were observed to the same extent in both groups (Table 2.5-2). Treatment-related mortality (TRM) was slightly higher in the Bu/Cy than in the TBI group (28% vs. 20%; p = 0.6) and was mainly due to interstitial pneumonia, GvHD and infections (see Table 2.5-3).

Relapse

Relapse was defined as haematologic relapse. After a median follow-up of 34 months (range: 5–65), 7 relapses (14%) were observed after a median of 12 months post transplantation (range: 3–50). All relapses occurred in the TBI group, but the median follow-up of the TBI group is longer than that of the Bu/Cy group (44 vs. 15 months). All patients with haematologic relapses

Table 2.5-3 Treatment-related mortality.

TRM	TBI/Cy	Bu/Cy
Interstitial pneumonia	0	2
GvHD	1	1
CMV disease	1	2
Sepsis/Bleeding	1	1
Aspergillus	2	1
Overall	5 (20%)	7 (28%)

received donor lymphocyte infusion. Three patients did not respond to DLI and 2 of these received a second transplant and are free of disease at the time of this evaluation. The third patient developed blast crisis and expired. Two patients died, of severe GvHD and sepsis, respectively. Two patients responded to DLI with complete disappearance of the bcr/abl transcript.

Overall survival and disease-free survival

After a median follow-up of 44 months (range: 34–65) in the TBI and of 15 months (range: 4–34) in the Bu/Cy group, the 3-year estimated overall survival (OS) is 72% (95% CI: 55–98%) for the TBI group and 70% (95% CI: 52–98%) for the Bu/Cy group (p = 0.7). The 3-year estimated disease-free survival (DFS) is 58% (95% CI: 39–77%) for the TBI and 70% (95% CI: 51–89%) for the BU/Cy regimen (p = 0.7) (Figs. 2.5-1 and 2.5-2). Age (< or > 40 years), incidence of acute or chronic GvHD or HLA-matched/mismatched donor did not affect outcome (data not shown). Patients transplanted with a CD34+ cell dose above 3.0 x 10^6/kg had a better 3-year estimated overall survival than did patients transplanted with a CD34+ cell dose below 3.0 x 10^6/kg (71% vs. 50%; p = 0.05).

Discussion

This is the first study comparing TBI with busulfan combined with cyclophosphamide as a preparative regimen in CML patients transplanted from an unrelated donor. TBI/cyclophosphamide is the most commonly used regimen in unrelated stem cell transplantation in patients with CML, because TBI may be necessary to achieve the degree of immunosuppression needed for engraftment since it has been shown that unrelated bone marrow transplantation is associated with a higher incidence of graft failure [3,15]. The combination of busulfan and cyclophosphamide was first described by SANTOS et al. [20]. Busulfan (16 mg/kg) and cyclophosphamide (200 mg/kg) provided an effective alternative to TBI plus cyclophosphamide in treatment of AML. Modification of this regimen by lowering the cyclophosphamide dose to 120 mg/kg appears to be equally effective and less toxic [24]. In an earlier study, the Bu/Cy regimen in unrelated bone marrow transplantation appeared to be associated with a higher incidence of graft failure than that reported after conditioning with TBI [8]. Recently, several single centre reports have demonstrated a low incidence of graft failure following conditioning with

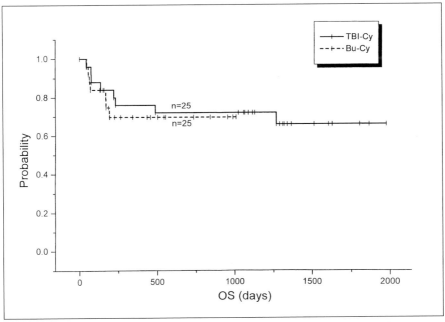

Figure 2.5-1 Overall survival of CML and unrelated stem cell transplantation after conditioning with TBI/Cy or BU/Cy.

busulfan and cyclophosphamide [11,19,23,24]. In our study all patients, including the 6 transplanted with one HLA mismatch, conditioned with the busulfan/cyclophosphamide regimen had rapid and sustained engraftment. There are two randomized trials of Bu/Cy *versus* TBI/Cy in related bone marrow transplantation for CML. The *French Society of Bone Marrow Grafting* found no significant differences with respect to overall and disease-free survival between the TBI/Cy and the Bu/Cy regimen, but they reported a higher incidence of graft failure for the Bu/Cy regimen and an increased risk of relapse after the TBI/Cy regimen, especially when fractionated TBI was given [6]. The other randomized trial from Seattle also reported no differences in disease-free and overall survival between the Bu/Cy and the TBI/Cy regimens, but the Bu/Cy regimen was better tolerated than was the TBI/Cy combination [5]. In a third retrospective study from the *Nordic Bone Marrow Transplantation Group* of TBI/Cy *versus* Bu/Cy in leukaemia patients a higher incidence of VOD (12% vs. 1%) and haemorrhagic cystitis (24% vs. 8%) was observed in the Bu/Cy arm. In the subgroup of CML patients no difference in overall and disease-free survival was seen [18]. In our study, the relapse rate was higher in the TBI/Cy group similar to the observation in the French study for related bone marrow transplantation. However, no definite conclusions should be drawn from this preliminary observation because of the different follow-ups in each arm (TBI/Cy 44 months, and Bu/Cy 15 months). At the time of this analysis, we found no differences in the 3-year estimated OS (72% vs. 70%) and the DFS (58% vs. 70%) between the TBI and the Bu/Cy group. We observed a trend for higher TRM in the Bu/Cy group (28%

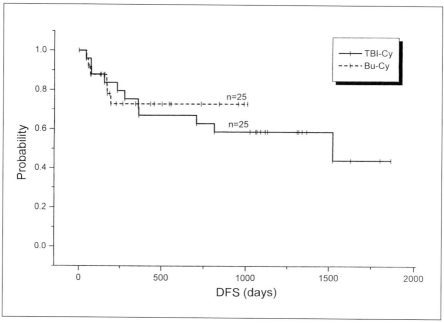

Figure 2.5-2 Disease-free survival of CML and unrelated stem cell transplantation after conditioning with TBI/Cy or BU/Cy.

vs. 20%) and more liver toxicity with Bu/Cy (p = 0.002). We further noted a higher incidence of haemorrhagic cystitis in the Bu/Cy group (32% vs. 8%), as was observed by the *Nordic Bone Marrow Transplantation Group*. Because of the oral formulation of busulfan and the differences in resorption, i.v. preparations of busulfan will facilitate its use, with more predictable serum levels and hence lower toxicity [1]. Chronic GvHD was more frequently seen in the Bu/Cy group (p = 0.02). HLA mismatch and PBSC as the stem cell source are known to be associated with a higher incidence of chronic GvHD, but even if these patients were censored, the incidence of cGvHD was twice as high in the Bu/Cy group (8 vs. 4 patients). This is in accordance with the findings of the *Nordic Bone Marrow Transplantation Group* [18], which also observed a higher incidence of cGvHD in related bone marrow transplantation after Bu/Cy than after TBI/Cy (45% vs. 35%, p = 0.04). The reasons for this observation are not clear, but the higher toxicity of the Bu/Cy regimen might have contributed to the higher incidence of cGvHD.

The outcome of unrelated bone marrow transplantation in CML has been adversely affected by age [8,9,15], HLA disparity, incidence of GvHD and the interval from diagnosis and transplantation [7,9]. In our study neither age (> 40 or < 40 years), incidence of acute or chronic GvHD or an HLA-matched/ mismatched donor affected outcome. However, the cell dose transplanted did affect overall survival but not the disease-free survival, which confirmed the importance of cell dose recently reported by several investigators [21]. The low incidence of severe GvHD and absence of graft failure in the entire study might be due to the incorporation of anti-thymocyte globulin in the preparative regimen, which has been shown to be effective in preventing severe GvHD and graft failure in HLA-matched and mismatched unrelated stem cell transplantation [12,26].

In conclusion, our preliminary results demonstrate that the anti-leukaemic effect of the Bu/Cy regimen seems to be at least as effective as the TBI/Cy combination in unrelated stem cell transplantation of CML patients without graft failure, but with a higher incidence of liver toxicity, haemorrhagic cystitis and chronic GvHD. Longer follow-up is necessary to determine late relapse rate and toxicity.

Acknowledgements

We thank the staff of the BMT unit for providing excellent care of our patients and the medical technicians for their excellent work in the BMT laboratory.

References

1. ANDERSSON, B.S., et al.: IV busulfan, cytoxan and allogeneic hematopoietic stem cell transplantation for advanced hematological malignancies. Bone Marrow Transplantation 23 (Suppl. 1) (1999) 223.
2. BEARMAN, S.I., et al.: Regimen-related toxicity in patients undergoing bone marrow transplantation. J Clin Oncol 6 (1988) 1562–1568.
3. BEATTY, P.G., et al.: The use of unrelated bone marrow donors in the treatment of chronic myelogenous leukemia: experience of four centers. Bone Marrow Transplantation 4 (1989) 287–290.
4. BERTZ, H., et al.: Busulfan/cyclophosphamide in volunteers unrelated donor (VUD) BMT: excellent feasibility and low incidence of treatment-related toxicity. Bone Marrow Transplantation 19 (1997) 1169–1173.
5. CLIFT, R.A., et al.: Marrow transplantation for chronic myeloid leukemia: a randomized study comparing cyclophosphamide and total body irradiation with busulfan and cyclophosphamide. Blood 84 (1994) 2036–2043.
6. DEVERGIE, A., et al.: Allogeneic Bone marrow transplantation for chronic myeloid leukemia in first chronic phase: a randomized trial of busulfan-cytoxan versus cytoxan-Total-body irradiation as preparative regimen: a report from the French Society of Bone Marrow Graft. Blood 85 (1995) 2263–2268.
7. DEVERGIE, A., et al.: For the Chronic Leukemia Working Party of the European Group of Blood and Marrow Transplantation. European results of matched unrelated bone marrow transplantation for chronic myeloid leukemia. Impact of HLA class II matching. Bone Marrow Transplantation 20 (1997) 11–19.
8. GRATWOHL, A., et al.: For the Chronic Leukemia Working party of the EBMT. Bone marrow transplantation for chronic myeloid leukemia: long-terms results. Bone Marrow Transplantation 12 (1993) 509–516.
9. HANSEN, J.A., et al.: Bone marrow transplants from unrelated donors for patients with chronic myeloid leukemia. N Engl J Med 338 (1998) 962–968.
10. KERNAN, N.A., et al.: Analysis of 462 transplantations from unrelated donors facilitated by the national marrow donor program. N Engl J Med (1993) 328: 593.
11. KLEIN, J.L., et al.: Bone marrow engraftment following unrelated donor transplantation utilizing busulfan and cyclophosphamide preparatory chemotherapy. Bone Marrow Transplantation 17 (1996) 479–483.
12. KRÖGER, N., et al.: Anti-human T-lymphocyte globulin (ATG) as part of the conditioning regimen in unrelated bone marrow transplantation of patients with CML in chronic or accelerated phase. Blood 92 (Suppl 1) (1998) 578.

13. MARK, D., *et al.*: Allogeneic bone marrow transplantation for chronic myeloid leukemia using sibling and volunteer unrelated donors: a comparison of complications in the first 2 years. Ann Intern Med 19 (1993) 207–214.

14. McDONALD, G.B., *et al.*: Veno-occlusive disease of the liver and multiorgan failure after bone marrow transplantation: a cohort study of 355 patients. Ann Intern Med 118 (1993) 255–267.

15. McGLAVE, P., *et al.*: Unrelated donor marrow transplantation for chronic myelogenous leukemia: Initial experience of the National Marrow Donor Program. Blood 81 (1993) 543.

16. METHA, J., *et al.*: Graft failure after bone marrow transplantation from unrelated donors using busulfan and cyclophosphamide for conditioning. Bone Marrow Transplantation 13 (1994) 583–587.

17. PRZEPIORKA, K.M., *et al.*: 1994 Consensus Conference on acute GvHD-grading. Bone Marrow Transplantation 15 (1995) 825–828.

18. RINGDEN, O., *et al.*: For the Nordic Bone Marrow Transplantation Group. A randomized trial comparing busulfan with total body irradiation as conditioning in allogeneic marrow transplant recipients with leukemia: a report from the Nordic Bone Marrow Transplantation Group. Blood 83 (1994) 2723–2730.

19. SAHEBI, F. *et al.*: Unrelated allogeneic bone marrow transplantation using high-dose busulfan and cyclophosphamide for preparative regimen. Bone Marrow Transplantation 17 (1996) 329–333.

20. SANTOS, G.W., *et al.*: Marrow transplantation for acute non-lymphomic leukemia after treatment with busulfan and cyclophosphamide. N Engl J Med 309 (1983) 1347–1353.

21. SIERRA, J., *et al.*: Transplantation of marrow cells from unrelated donors for treatment of high-risk acute leukemia: the effect of leukemia burden, donor HLA-matching and marrow cell dose. Blood 89 (1997) 4226–4235.

22. SPENCER, A., *et al.*: Bone marrow transplantation for chronic myeloid leukemia with volunteer unrelated donors using ex vivo or in vivo T-cell depletion: major prognostic impact of HLA class I identity between donor and recipient. Blood 86 (1995) 3590–3597.

23. TOPOLSKY, D., *et al.*: Unrelated donor bone marrow transplantation without T cell depletion using a chemotherapy only conditioning regimen. Low incidence of failed engraftment and severe acute GvHD. Bone Marrow Transplantation 17 (1996) 549–554.

24. TUTSCHKA, P.J., *et al*: Bone marrow transplantation for leukemia following new busulfan and cyclophosphamide regime. Blood 70 (1987) 1382–88.

25. ZANDER, A.R., *et al.*: Use of a five-agent GvHD prevention regimen in recipients of unrelated donor marrow. Bone Marrow Transplantation 23 (1999) 889–893.

26. ZANDER, A.R. *et al.*: Bone marrow transplantation from mismatched unrelated donors. Bone Marrow Transplantation 25 (Suppl 1) (2000) 36.

2.6 Current Concepts in Allogeneic and Autologous Stem Cell Transplantation for Chronic Lymphocytic Leukaemia

Dreger, P.

2nd Dept. of Medicine, University of Kiel, Germany

Supported by the José-Carreras-Leukämie-Stiftung (DJCLS-R16)

Summary

Allogeneic and autologous stem cell transplantation (SCT) are increasingly considered for treatment of patients with chronic lymphocytic leukaemia (CLL). In order to assess the potential therapeutic value of SCT for CLL, the present article aims at answering the following crucial questions: (1) Is SCT a curative treatment? (2) Does SCT improve the dismal prognosis of poor-risk CLL? (3) Do risk factors exist which are useful for defining prognostic groups in terms of feasibility and post-transplant outcome? The efficacy of auto-SCT relies exclusively on the cytotoxic therapy administered. To date, there is only limited hope that autotransplantation can cure the disease, even in this favourable subgroup. Nevertheless, the results of the published series suggest that auto-SCT is capable of improving the prognosis of CLL with defined poor-risk features. Favourable conditions for successful autografting are less advanced disease, a sufficient remission status at SCT and use of a TBI-containing high-dose regimen. The crucial anti-leukaemic principle of allo-SCT consists in the immune-mediated GvL effects conferred with the graft. The GvL activity should be responsible for the fact that allografting seems to be a curative treatment for at least a subset of poor-risk patients. As long as allo-SCT in CLL is, however, still associated with an excessively high treatment-related mortality, only selected patients with advanced poor-risk disease should be considered for allografting. The development of conditioning regimens with reduced intensity may allow the extension of the indications of allogeneic SCT for CLL in the near future.

Allogeneic and autologous stem cell transplantation (SCT) are increasingly considered for treatment of patients with chronic lymphocytic leukaemia (CLL). In order to assess the potential therapeutic value of SCT for CLL, the present article reviews the most important clinical studies in this field, thereby attempting to answer the following crucial questions for both allo- and auto-SCT: (1) Is SCT a curative treatment? (2) Does SCT improve the dismal prognosis of poor-risk CLL? (3) Do risk factors exist which are useful for defining prognostic groups in terms of feasibility and post-transplant outcome?

Autologous stem cell transplantation

To date, only four studies on autologous SCT for CLL are available which comprise sufficiently large patient numbers with informative analyses of

Table 2.6-1 Autologous SCT in CLL.

Trial	EBMT [3]	Int. Project [8]	Kiel [4]	GCLLSG
Trial type	Registry data, retrospective	Registry data, retrospective	Single centre prospective	Single centre prospective
n	370	107	77	105
TRM	10%	7%	4%	5%
2-y-EFS	no	69%	87%	no
4-y-EFS	no	37%	69%	no
2-y-OS	82%	83%	94%	88%*
4-y-OS	69%	65%	94%	no
Plateau	no	no	no	no

TRM = treatment-related mortality
2-y-EFS = event-free survival 2 years post SCT
2-y-OS = overall survival 2 years post SCT
* survival of all patients included 2 years after start of treatment (intent-to-transplant analysis)

prognostic factors to allow an approach to these three critical issues: The recent update of the CLL database of the *European Group for Blood and Marrow Transplantation* (EBMT) [3], the *International Project on CLL Transplants* [8], the 2nd interim analysis of the CLL3 study of the *German CLL Study Group* (to be published), and the series from Kiel [4].

Is autologous SCT a curative treatment?

As summarized in Table 2.6-1, all of these four studies are characterized by a low treatment-related mortality (TRM) on the one hand and the lack of a plateau in the event- or relapse-free survival curves on the other hand. The fact that patients continue to relapse up to 5 years post transplant, at least, does not support the hypothesis that autografting can be curative in certain subsets of patients with CLL.

Another argument against the curative potential of auto-SCT comes from results of the molecular follow-up of the patients from the Kiel series: Allele-specific PCR amplification of the complementary determining region 3 of the IgH gene (ASO CDR3 PCR) detected residual disease in at least two follow-up samples in 28 of 35 cases (80%) with specific CDR3 primers available, although more than half of the patients with a positive ASO PCR had no evidence of disease by consensus primer PCR, flow cytometry, or clinical assessment. Molecular persistence or recurrence of CLL post transplant was not correlated with Binet stage. This implies that complete disease eradication was not possible by this intensive approach in the vast majority of patients, even though the Kiel protocol included highly effective tools for *in-vivo* and *ex-vivo* CLL cell depletion and focused on individuals with early (though poor-risk) disease. Taken together, there is limited hope that CLL can be cured by standard myeloablative therapy with reinfusion of *ex-vivo* B-cell depleted autografts alone.

Does autologous SCT improve the prognosis of patients with CLL?

A reliable evaluation of the impact of SCT on the prognosis of CLL requires prospectively randomized studies comparing autografting with conventional

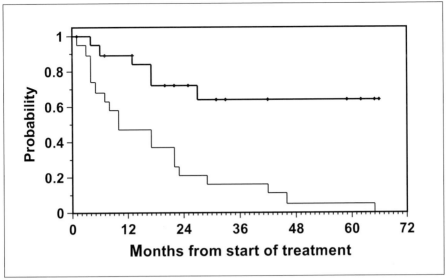

Figure 2.6-1 Freedom from treatment failure (FFTF) in the patients who underwent salvage SCT.
Thin line = FFTF after the last conventional regimen prior to SCT attempt
Bold line = FFTF after start of high-dose protocol (by intention-to-treat)

palliative treatment. As such studies are completely lacking to date, the possible prognostic benefit of SCT can only be roughly extrapolated from the results of the published single-arm series. These studies, however, usually suffer from patient heterogeneity and selection bias, and, thus, can hardly be compared with the generally accepted results of conventional therapy. With these limitations in mind, the Barcelona group plotted the overall survival of the advanced-stage patients from the International Project against the overall survival of conventionally-treated but otherwise similar patients from their own database, and found a significant prognostic advantage for auto-SCT (Jordi ESTEVE, personal communication). In the Kiel series, we analysed the 19 patients in whom autografting was attempted as part of a second-line strategy. In these 19 individuals, freedom from treatment failure (FFTF) post mobilization (= SCT attempt) was compared to FFTF after the last conventional regimen prior to mobilization. It became apparent that FFTF after SCT attempt was much longer than after the last standard chemotherapy (median FFTF 10 months vs. not reached, p = 0.0002; Fig. 2.6-1), implying that SCT allows more efficient tumour control than conventional treatment. Taken together, although the results of the published trials are promising, data illustrating a clear-cut therapeutic benefit of autografting in CLL are still very sparse, and the results of the ongoing prospective studies have to be awaited.

Are there prognostic factors predicting the outcome after autologous SCT?

Prognostic factor analyses are important to identify subgroups of patients who are most likely to benefit from SCT, and to define the optimum timing of SCT.

Table 2.6-2 Prognostic factor analysis for post transplant outcome in autologous SCT in CLL.

Trial	EBMT	Int. Project	Kiel	GCLLSG
Method	Cox analysis	Cox analysis	log rank test	log rank test
Endpoint	relapse incidence	disease-free survival	molecular clonality	molecular clonality
Variables analysed	age, sex, time from diagnosis, fludarabine treatment, status at SCT purging, TBI	fludarabine response, time from diagnosis, pretreatment, status at SCT, purging, TBI	age, sex, time from diagnosis, pretreatment, lymphocyte count, Binet stage	caryotype, time from diagnosis, pretreatment, lymphocyte count, Binet stage, status at SCT
Favourable variables	CR at SCT, < 36 mos. from diagn.,TBI yes	CR at SCT	lymphocytes < 50G/l	CR at SCT, caryotype other than del 11q-

TBI = total body irradiation
CR = complete remission

Possible explanatory variables predicting for the success of autografting can be divided into three groups: (i) Course-related risk factors are those which develop as the disease continues (e.g. stage, time from diagnosis, intensity of pretreatment, timing of transplant). Their prognostic impact may be bypassed by early transplant. (ii) Biological risk factors are determined by genuine biological features of the tumour clone and cannot necessarily be eliminated by early timing of transplant (e.g. age, sex, lymphocyte count, lymphocyte doubling time, cytogenetics, mutational status).

(iii) Technical risk factors are related to the transplant procedure itself and, thus, can be influenced (e.g. source of stem cells, purging, high-dose regimen, remission status at transplant). Prognostic factor analyses are available for all four studies mentioned. Their results are listed in Table 2.6-2 and can be summarized as follows: As far as analysed, biological risk factors, such as lymphocyte count and adverse cytogenetics, are associated with an inferior post transplant outcome. Among the technical risk factors, insufficient remission at SCT and, possibly, the use of high-dose regimens not containing total body irradiation (TBI) might have an adverse influence, whereas course-related factors, such as stage and time from diagnosis, appear to be less important.

Another issue is the question of pretransplant failure, i.e. which patients scheduled for transplant cannot undergo autografting due to lack of a suitable graft or a sufficient response. This question has been addressed in the prospective Kiel and GCLLSG trials. In both series, about one fifth of all patients considered for transplant experienced pretransplant failure. A history of Binet stage C disease was the predominant factor predicting for poor pretransplant outcome, as illustrated by a failure probability of 36% and 58%, respectively, in the Kiel and CLL3 studies.

Taking into account their preliminary character, these analyses support the requirement of a sufficient remission status at SCT as well as the use of TBI. Furthermore, they suggest that randomized trials on SCT might be best performed in a salvage setting, since the results of conventional second-line treatment in CLL are poor, whereas the outcome after autografting is encouraging and does not appear to be very much different between patients with early and advanced disease, respectively. Thus, the possible benefits of SCT will emerge easier and faster if studied as second-line treatment. Whether this, on the other side, questions the justification of further trials on early transplant remains highly debatable: Almost every patient with poor-risk features will progress to a symptomatic stage and, ultimately, fulfil the criteria for SCT. Delaying high-dose therapy until advanced stage or need for salvage treatment, however, implies that many patients will never receive an autograft due to mobilization failure and resistant disease.

Allogeneic stem cell transplantation

Allogeneic SCT is a treatment approach which is fundamentally different from autologous transplantation, particularly in the context of indolent diseases such as CLL. Whereas efficacy (and complications) of autografting rely exclusively on the cytotoxic therapy administered, the crucial anti-leukaemic principle of allotransplantation appears to be the immune-mediated anti-host activities conferred with the graft (GvL effects). Accordingly, autologous SCT adds nothing else than intensity (and perhaps a radiotherapeutic component) to conventional treatment. For this reason, the toxicity of autotransplantation is nowadays only slightly higher than that of intensive conventional chemo-therapeutic regimens, but its capacity for complete eradication of resistant CLL clones seems to be limited, too. On the other hand, allogeneic transplantation introduces the entirely different modality of cellular immune therapy, which appears to be responsible for its superior anti-leukaemic activity as well as for its considerably higher toxicity.

Is allogeneic SCT a curative treatment?

Three larger series on allogeneic SCT for CLL have been published and are summarized in Table 2.6-3 [5,7,9]. All three studies are characterized by a high TRM on the one hand and a very low relapse incidence on the other hand: The

Table 2.6-3 Allogeneic SCT in CLL.

Trial	EBMT [7]	Omaha [9]	MD Anderson [5]
Trial type	registry data, retrospective	single centre retrospective	single centre retrospective
n	134	23	15
TRM	40%	30%	57%
4-y-OS	54%	62%	27%
Plateau	yes	yes	yes

TRM = treatment-related mortality
2-y-EFS = event-free survival 2 years post SCT
2-y-OS = overall survival 2 years post SCT
* survival of all patients included 2 years after start of treatment (intent-to-transplant analysis)

survival curves appear to approach a plateau in the long term, suggesting that allotransplantation may have curative potential in this disease. The superior tumour control provided by allografting in comparison to autografting suggests a pronounced susceptibility of CLL to GVL effects.

Another line of evidence for the presence of GVL activity and, thus, curative potential of allografting in CLL comes from the documented efficacy of donor lymphocyte infusions and the fact that CLL cells persisting after dose-reduced conditioning for allogeneic SCT disappear with the onset of chronic graft-versus-host disease [1].

Does allogeneic SCT improve the prognosis of patients with CLL?

In spite of the low relapse rate, the survival after allo-SCT is significantly lower than after autologous SCT, at least during the first 4 years. The reason for this is the high toxicity associated with allografting for this particular indication. Even in well experienced centres, the TRM of allogeneic SCT in patients with CLL is reported to be up to 50% (Table 2.6-3). The causes of these detrimental results are not completely clear, but patient age, selection of poor-risk patients with advanced disease and extensive pretreatment, and the CLL-associated incompetence of the immune system may all contribute to the high TRM observed. The recent development of conditioning regimens with reduced intensity may help to improve the tolerability of allo-SCT in CLL without affecting its GvL activities [2,4].

In conclusion, at the present time allo-SCT in CLL should be restricted to symptomatic patients with very high-risk disease, such as those with unfavourable cytogenetics, early relapse after purine analogues, or failure of autografting. In these subgroups, the considerable risk of TRM should be more than outweighed by the prognostic improvement due to the effective disease control provided by allogeneic SCT.

Are there prognostic factors predicting the outcome after allogeneic SCT?

Conclusive prognostic factor analyses for identifying subgroups of patients who are most likely to benefit from allogeneic SCT for CLL are not available to date.

Conclusions and perspectives

Autologous and allogeneic stem cell transplantation appear to be fundamentally different treatment modalities for patients with CLL.

Autologous transplantation

The efficacy of auto-SCT relies exclusively on the cytotoxic therapy administered. With appropriate supportive care, it is safe and can induce long-lasting clinical and molecular remissions. Feasibility of autologous SCT appears to be best early during the course of the disease, but there is only limited hope that autotransplantation can cure the disease even in this favourable subgroup. Nevertheless, the results of the published series suggest that auto-SCT is capable of improving the prognosis of CLL with defined poor-risk features. Favourable

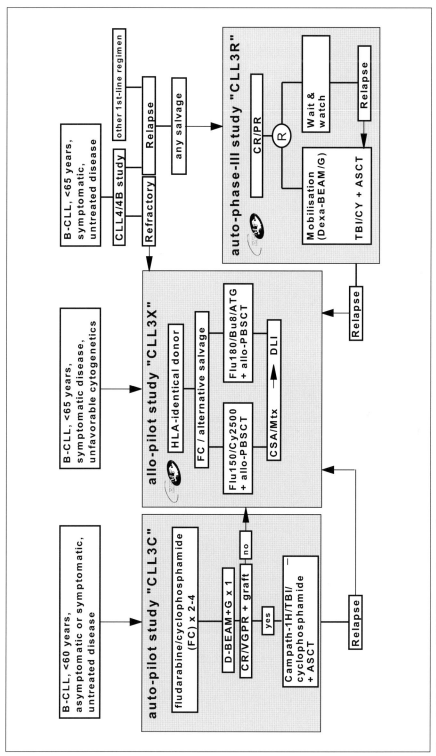

Figure 2.6-2 Current GCLLSG transplant studies.

conditions for successful autografting are: less advanced disease, a sufficient remission status at SCT and use of a TBI-containing high-dose regimen. Since post transplant outcome does not appear to be very much different between patients with first-line and salvage SCT, respectively, randomized trials on auto-SCT might be best performed in a salvage setting, where the results of conventional second-line treatment in CLL are poor, and, thus, the possible benefits of SCT are likely to emerge easier and faster. Such a trial has been started recently as a combined effort of the EBMT and the GCLLSG (*CLL3R* trial of the GCLLSG). Given the excellent feasibility of auto-SCT in early (but not in advanced) stages, further refinement of the procedure towards cure by implementing additional modalities, such as monoclonal antibodies, should focus on early patients. Along this line the GCLLSG *CLL3C trial* has been designed. The objective of this recently launched phase-II study is to investigate the safety and feasibility of the addition of CAMPATH-1H to the high-dose regimen for autologous SCT in patients with poor-risk CLL (Fig. 2.6-2).

Allotransplantation

The crucial anti-leukaemic principle of allotransplantation in CLL consists in the immune-mediated GVL effects conferred with the graft. The GVL activity should be responsible for the better disease control observed. Thus, allografting seems to be a curative treatment for at least a subset of poor-risk patients. However, as long as allo-SCT in CLL is still associated with an excessively high TRM, only selected patients with advanced poor-risk disease and low probability of successful auto-SCT should be considered for allografting. The development of conditioning regimens with reduced intensity may allow the extension of the indications of allogeneic SCT for CLL in the near future. To this end, the GCLLSG runs the EBMT-approved *CLL3X* trial, which studies fludarabine-based conditioning regimens in patients with very-high-risk CLL (Figure 2.6-2).

Taken together, we believe that autologous transplantation is preferable for patients with early or sensitive disease. Selected patients with advanced poor-risk disease and low probability of successful auto-SCT should be considered for allografting. It must, however, be kept in mind that both autologous and allogeneic stem cell transplantation are still experimental procedures which should not be performed outside of approved clinical trials.

References

1. DREGER, P., et al.: Reduced-intensity allogeneic stem cell transplantation as salvage treatment for patients with indolent lymphoma after failure of autologous SCT. Bone Marrow Transplant 26(2000):1361–1362.
2. DREGER, P., et al.: Allogeneic stem cell transplantation for poor-risk CLL using fludarabine/cyclophosphamide (FC) conditioning. Bone Marrow Transplant 27(2001):S37 (Abstract).
3. DREGER, P., et al.: Prognostic factors for survival after autologous stem cell transplantation for chronic lymphocytic leukemia (CLL): the EBMT experience. Blood 96(2000a):482a (Abstract).
4. DREGER, P., et al.: Feasibility and efficacy of early autologous stem cell transplantation for poor-risk CLL. Blood 96 Suppl.1(2000b):483a (Abstract).

5. KHOURI, I., *et al.*: Allogeneic blood or marrow transplantation for chronic lymphocytic leukaemia: timing of transplantation and potential effect of fludarabine on acute graft-versus-host disease. Br J Haematol 97(1997):466–473.

6. KHOURI, I.F., *et al.*: Transplant-lite: induction of graft-versus-malignancy using fludarabine-based nonablative chemotherapy and allogeneic blood progenitor-cell transplantation as treatment for lymphoid malignancies. J Clin Oncol 16(1998):2817–2824.

7. MICHALLET, M., *et al.*: Allotransplants and autotransplants in CLL. Bone Marrow Transplant 23 Suppl.1(1999):S53 (Abstract).

8. MONTSERRAT, E., *et al.*: Autologous stem cell transplantation for CLL: analysis of the impact on overall survival in 107 patients from The International Project for CLL/transplants. Blood 94 Suppl.1(1999):397a.

9. PAVLETIC, Z.S., *et al.*: Outcome of allogeneic stem cell transplantation for B cell chronic lymphocytic leukemia. Bone Marrow Transplant 25(2000):717–722.

Part Three
Management of Graft-versus-Host Disease

3.1 GvHD Prophylaxis with Anti-Thymocyte Globulin in Recipients of Matched Unrelated Donor Transplants for Chronic Myelogenous Leukaemia: A Retrospective Analysis

Zander[1]*, A. R., N. Kröger[1], H. J. Kolb[2], J. Finke[3], T. Zabelina[1], M. Schleuning[2], D. W. Beelen[4], R. Schwerdtfeger[5], H. Baurmann[5], M. Bornhäuser[6], G. Ehninger[6], A. Fauser[7], M. Kiehl[7], R. Trenschel[4], U. W. Schäfer[4]

[1] Bone Marrow Transplantation Centre, University Hospital, Hamburg-Eppendorf, [2] Med. Clinic 3, Bone Marrow Transplantation Unit, University Hospital, Munich, [3] Dept. of Medicine, University Hospital, Freiburg, [4] Dept. of Bone Marrow Transplantation, University Hospital, Essen, [5] German Clinic for Diagnostic, Centre of Bone Marrow Transplantation, Wiesbaden, [6] Medical Clinic 1, University Hospital, Dresden, [7] Clinic for Bone Marrow Transplantation, Idar-Oberstein, Germany

* To whom correspondence should be addressed (zander@uke.uni-hamburg.de)

Summary

A retrospective analysis was carried out in three groups of patients treated with either anti-thymocytes globulin (ATG) using two preparations, from Fresenius (n = 80, average 90 mg/kg BW) and from Merieux (n = 66, average 10 mg/kg BW), or no ATG, as a control group (n = 188). The group which received ATG revealed superior survival at 3 years (72% vs. 66% vs. 57%), had decreased severe GvHD III–IV (9% vs. 35% vs. 22%), and decreased TRM (24% vs. 27% vs. 37%) with close to identical disease-free survival DFS of 60% vs. 60% vs. 55%. A prospective randomized study is needed to evaluate the role of ATG in HSCT.

Introduction

Matched unrelated donor transplant patients have an increased risk of severe graft-versus-host disease and transplant-related mortality [1–9]. ATG, as part of the conditioning regimen, resulted in a low rate of severe GvHD without obvious increase of relapse-rate and infection [4,7,11]. ATG preparations have been reported to vary in their side effects [2,4,7].

We conducted a retrospective analysis in CML patients from seven German *bone marrow transplantation centres* forming three groups, one which had been treated with ATG Fresenius S (n = 80, average 90 mg/kg BW; range 20–90 mg/kg), a second one with Thymoglobuline Merieux (n = 66, average 10 mg/kg BW; range 5–20 mg/kg) and the third one which received no ATG (n = 188).

Material and methods

A total of 146 patients had been treated with ATG: 80, with ATG-Fresenius, and 66, with Thymoglobuline Merieux; 188 patients had not received ATG. The patients characteristics are shown in Table 3.1-1. Comparing ATG vs. non-ATG, neither median age, nor sex distribution of patients, nor HLA match vs.

Table 3.1-1 Patient characteristics.

	ATG	Non ATG	p-value
Number of patients	146	188	
Median age	36 (r.: 6-58)	38 (r.: 18-58)	n.s.
Sex of patients (m:f)	89 : 57	118 : 70	n.s.
Cell source (BM:PBSC)	128 : 18 (12%)	133 : 55 (29%)	< 0.01
HLA match/mismatch	121 : 25 (17%)	143 : 45 (24%)	n.s.
Conditioning: TBI/Cy	25	147	
Bu/Cy	121	41	
CMV status: negative	86	107	n.s.
positive	60	81	n.s.
Median follow-up (days)	798 (9-2219)	899 (57-3342)	n.s.

mismatch, nor CMV status or median follow-up differ significantly between the two groups. In the two groups, a significant difference could be seen in the rate (bone marrow cells vs. PBSC) used as a cell source for transplantation. TBI occurred more frequently in the non-ATG group.

HLA typing and donor matching

HLA-A and B antigens were typed by serologic methods [3,6]. HLA-DRB1 and HLA-DQB1 alleles were determined by sequence-specific oligonucleotide probes. Donors were required to match the recipients for serologically defined HLA-A and B antigens as well as HLA-DRB1 and DQB1 alleles. In every patient a pre-transplantation lymphocyte cross-match (patient sera vs. donor cells) was performed. The total of HLA mismatches (A, B, DRB1,DQB1) amounted to 70.

Stem cell source

Eighteen out of 146 patients in the ATG group and 55 out of 188 in the non-ATG group received PBSC. The CMV status of recipients prior to transplant was 86 pos. vs. 146 neg. in the ATG group and 107 pos. vs. 188 neg. in the non-ATG group.

Transplant preparative regimens

The conditioning consisted in a combination of either total body irradiation/cyclophosphamide or busulfan/cyclophosphamide. There was an unequal distribution of conditioning regimens with 25/146 TBI conditioning in the ATG group versus 147/188 TBI conditioning in the non-ATG group.

GvHD prophylaxis and treatment

GvHD prophylaxis consisting of cyclosporine A (3 mg/kg BW) was given from day –1 with several reductions for six months post transplant. The dose of cyclosporine A was adjusted to lower levels, tapered and discontinued at day 180. Methotrexate (10 mg/m²) was given on days 1, 3 and 6 in the ATG group and on day 11 in the non-ATG group.

Antithymocyte globulin (Fresenius Bad Homburg, Germany) was given to 80 patients with an average dose of 30 mg/kg/day on day –3, –2, –1. Thymo-globuline was given in an average dose of 10 mg/kg (range 5–20 mg/kg BW) distributed over 4 days. Standard criteria were used for the diagnosis of acute and chronic graft-versus-host disease [10]. Acute GvHD (II–IV) was treated with high-dose steroids and extensive chronic GvHD with cyclosporine A and steroids, as well as mycophenolate mofetil. Chronic GvHD was evaluated in patients who survived at least 80 days with sustained engraftment.

Supportive care

All patients were nursed in single rooms with HEPA-filtered air. Antibiotic, antifungal, and antiviral prophylaxis was given according to the standards of the transplant centre. Blood products were irradiated prior to infusion. Peripheral blood products all originated from CMV-negative donors. Monitoring of blood and urine for CMV antigen by PCR, and short term culture were carried out weekly or bi-weekly. In case of recurring detection, antiviral therapy with ganciclovir was initiated.

Statistical methods

Statistical analysis was performed using a WIN-STAT software (Kalmia Co., Inc., Cambridge, MA, USA). Survival curves for disease-free survival and overall survival were estimated by the Kaplan-Meier method.

Results

Table 3.1-2 shows the results for the 3 groups. Graft-failure occurred in 1% in the ATG group, in 6% in the thymoglobulin group, and in 2% in the non-ATG group. Acute GvHD II–IV was seen in 27%, 55% and 43%, respectively. Transplant-related mortality was 24%, 29% and 37% and the overall survival was 72%, 66% and 57%.

When the two ATG groups were combined, ATG showed a significantly faster engraftment, i.e. day 16 vs. day 20 (p = < 0,001) (see Table 3.1-3). No difference in the graft-failure rate could be detected. Acute GvHD II–V occurred in 62% vs. 77% (p = 0,003), and transplant-related mortality in 26% vs. 69% (p = 0,04). The relapse rate (10% vs. 5%) was not significant.

Table 3.1-2 Results related to ATG use (Fresenius vs. Merieux vs. non-ATG).

	ATG-Fresenius n = 80	ATG-Merieux n = 66	non-ATG n = 188
Engraftment	15 (10–24)	18 (11–32)	20 (8–38)
Graft-failure	1 (1%)	4 (6%)	4 (2%)
aGvHD II–IV	27%	55%	43%
aGvHD III–IV	9%	35%	22%
cGvHD overall	54%	54%	66%
cGvHD ext.	29%	18%	20%
Relapse rate	11%	9%	5%
TRM	24%	29%	37%
OS 3 years	72%	65%	57%
DFS	60%	57%	55%

Table 3.1-3 Results.

	ATG	non-ATG	p-value
Engraftment L > 1.0	16 (10–32)	20 (8–38)	< 0.001
Graft-failure	5 (3%)	4 (2%)	n.s.
aGvHD	88 (62%)	141 (77%)	0.003
cGvHD overall	67 (54%)	108 (66%)	0.03
TRM	38 (26%)	69 (37%)	0.04
Relapse	15 (10%)	10 (5%)	n.s.

Side effects of ATG

Main side effects were fever, chills, flush and one case of anaphylactic reaction with bronchospasm and hypertension responding to administration of cortico-steroids.

Survival

The overall survival at 3 years was 67% vs. 57% (p = 0,09) in favour of ATG. Recipients of HLA-mismatched bone marrow in the ATG group had the same overall survival as the recipients of HLA-matched stem cell grafts, whereas the overall survival of recipients of HLA-mismatched grafts in the non-ATG group was worse than that of the HLA-matched recipients.

Discussion

In our retrospective analysis, ATG did not lead to an increased graft rejection rate nor to an increased rate of secondary lymphomas. There was a trend towards a higher relapse rate in the ATG group. The recipient's CMV status predicted for overall survival, event-free survival and TRM. Conditioning with TBI and cyclophosphamide vs. busulfan and cyclophosphamide did not show a difference in outcome. As to age, less than 40 vs. more than 40 years was not a significant factor for overall survival.

With the use of ATG we observed no difference in the outcome of mismatched and matched unrelated donor transplant recipients in contrast to the non-ATG group. The retrospective data compare favourably with reports of unrelated donor transplant previously published [3, 6].

The reduction of the incidence of acute and chronic GvHD by the administration of ATG has been documented by several groups with several ATG preparations [4,7,10]. The ATG preparations might vary significantly in their degree of immunosuppression and side effects.

In this retrospective analysis, the ATG groups were too small to look for differences in the clinical outcome. ATG, as part of the preparative regimen in matched unrelated stem cell transplantation, reduces the risk of transplant-related mortality and acute GvHD without an obvious increase of relapse or severe infections. Further studies are necessary to optimize the dose for unrelated donor transplantation. A prospective randomized study is needed, in order to determine the definite role of ATG in haemopoietic stem cell transplantation.

References

1. ANASETTI, C., *et al.*: Effect of HLA incompatibility on graft-versus-host disease, relapse, and survival after marrow transplantation for patients with leukemia and lymphoma. Hum Immunol 29 (1990) 79.
2. BATIA, S., *et al.*: Malignant neoplasms following bone marrow transplantation. Blood 87 (1996) 3633–3639.
3. BEATTY, P.G., *et al.*: Marrow transplantation from related donors other than HLA-identical siblings. N Engl J Med 313 (19985) 765.
4. FINKE, J., *et al.*: Allogeneic bone marrow transplantation from unrelated donors using in vivo anti-T-cell globulin. British Journal of Haematology 111 (2000) (1) 303–313.
5. HANSEN, J.A., *et al.*: Bone marrow transplants from unrelated donors for patients with chronic myeloid leukemia. N Engl J Med 338 (1998) 962.
6. KERNAN, N.A., *et al.*: Analysis of 462 transplantations from unrelated donors facilitated by the national marrow donor program. N Engl J Med 328 (1993) 593.
7. KRÖGER, N., *et al.*: Patient cytomegalovirus seropositivity with or without reactivation as the most important prognostic factor for survival and treatment-related mortality in stem cell transplantation form unrelated donors using pretransplant in vivo T-cell depletion with anti-thymocyte globulin. British Journal of Hematology 113 (2001) 1–13 (in press).
8. MCGLAVE, P., *et al.*: Unrelated donor marrow transplantation for chronic myelogenous leukemia: initial experience of the National Marrow Donor Program. Blood 81 (1993) 543.
9. NADEMANEE A., *et al.*: The outcome of matched unrelated donor bone marrow transplantation in patients with hematologic malignancies using molecular typing for donor selection and graft-versus-host disease prophylaxis regimen of cyclosporine, methotrexate, and prednisone. Blood 86 (1995) 1228.
10. PRZEPIORKA, K.M., *et al.*: Consensus Conference on acute GvHD-grading. Bone Marrow Transplantation 15 (1995) 825–828.
11. ZANDER, A.R., *et al.*: Use of a five-agent GvHD prevention regimen in recipients of unrelated donor marrow. Bone Marrow Transplantation 23 (1999) 889–893.

3.2 Low Treatment-Related Mortality Following Allografting in Advanced Multiple Myeloma after an Intensified Conditioning Regimen and Anti-Thymocyte Globulin for GvHD Prevention

Kröger[1]*, N., G. Derigs[2], H. Wandt[3], K. Schäfer-Eckart[3], G. Wittkowsky[4], R. Kuse[4] , J. Casper[5], W. Krüger[1], T. Zabelina[1], H. Renges[1], H. Kabisch[1], A. Krüll[6], H. Einsele[7], A. R. Zander[1]

[1] Bone Marrow Transplantation and [6] Dept. of Radiotherapy, Eppendorf University Hospital, Hamburg, [2] University Hospital, Mainz, [3] Städt. Klinikum, Nürnberg, [4] Dept. of Haematology, A. K. St. Georg, Hamburg, [5] University Hospital, Rostock, [7] University Hospital, Tübingen, Germany

* To whom correspondence should be addressed (nkroeger@uke.uni-hamburg.de)

Summary

In order to reduce the incidence of severe graft-versus-host disease (GvHD), and lower the treatment-related mortality (TRM) in allogeneic stem cell transplantation from HLA-identical siblings in patients with multiple myeloma, we incorporated anti-thymocyte globulin in the conditioning regimen of 12 patients. The conditioning regimen consisted of modified total body irradiation, busulfan and cyclophosphamide or busulfan and cyclophosphamide.

The median age was 44 years (range 29–53) and the median time from diagnosis to transplant was 12 months (range 6–56). The stem cell source was bone marrow in 10 and peripheral blood stem cells in 2 patients. Grade II–IV acute GvHD occurred in 3 patients (27%). Severe grade III and IV GvHD developed in only 1 patient. Major toxicity was mucositis. Grade II, according to the Bearman score, was observed in 10 patients, whereas 2 patients experienced grade III, requiring prophylactic intubation. One patient died of severe GvHD grade IV, and one patient developed multi-organ failure on day +13, resulting in a TRM of 17%. A complete response in surviving patients after allogeneic transplantation was seen in 4 (40%), and PR in 6 (60%) patients. Two of the patients with PR received a donor lymphocyte infusion (DLI), for further tumour reduction, 8 and 14 months after stem cell transplantation, and converted to CR, which increased the rate of CR to 60%. After a median follow-up of 25 months (range 5–62), no patient with CR after allogeneic transplantation relapsed during follow-up, while 3 out of 4 patients with PR experienced tumour progression within 3 years (p = 0.07). The estimated overall survival at three years for all patients is 83 percent (CI 95%: 68%–98%). The estimated progression-free survival at three years is 61 percent (CI 95%: 32%–90%). These results suggest that including anti-thymocyte globulin may prevent severe GvHD without obvious increase of relapse. DLI should be given to patients with incomplete response after transplantation, in order to enhance the rate of complete remissions, thereby assuring a long-term disease-free status.

Introduction

Allogeneic stem cell transplantation may cure patients with multiple myeloma. In a retrospective study of the EBMT, 42% of the patients are disease-free 5 years after allogeneic transplantation [8]. The advantage of allogeneic stem cells over autologous stem cells is a direct anti-tumour activity due to the graft-versus-myeloma effect of allogeneic immunocompetent T-cells [13,20,21]. However, the transplant-related morbidity and mortality attained 40%, resulting in a change for the worse when compared to autologous transplantation from a retro-spective case-matched study [4], albeit a lower progression rate. Therefore, efforts were made to better these results by improving the selection of patients, ameliorating the timing of transplant [18], using PBSC as stem cell source [14], and decreasing the transplant-related mortality by using more effective methods to prevent severe graft-versus-host disease [1,19]. Recently, the EBMT registry reported a lower transplant-related mortality, i.e. 20%, for patients transplanted after 1995 [99]. To reduce treatment-related mortality and retain anti-tumour efficacy, we investigated *in vivo* T-cell depletion with anti-thymocyte globulin in patients with multiple myeloma, as part of the conditioning regimen, consisting of total marrow irradiation, busulfan and cyclophosphamide versus busulfan/cyclophosphamide alone prior to allogeneic stem cell transplantation with HLA-identical siblings. Comparable data showed that ATG, as part of the conditioning regimen, resulted in a low incidence of severe acute and chronic GvHD in unrelated bone marrow transplantation without apparent increase in the relapse rate [20].

Patients and methods

Characteristics

Between 1995 and 2000, 12 patients with a median age of 44 years (range 29–53) were enrolled in the protocol. A written informed consent was received from each patient, and the study was approved by the local Ethics Committee. Major inclusion criteria were age below 55 years, disease stage II or III and the presence of an HLA-identical sibling as donor. There were 9 male and 3 female patients. All patients had shown at least a minor response to preceding induction chemotherapy. Six out of 12 patients had been previously subjected to radiation therapy, excluding 3 of them from total marrow irradiation. The median β_2-microglobulin serum level at diagnosis was 2.5 mg/dl (range 1.7–7.6). The median time from diagnosis to transplant was 12 months (range 6–56). The characteristics of the patients are shown in Table 3.2-1.

Conditioning

In 9 patients, conditioning was achieved by total-marrow irradiation applying 900 cGy given over three days in 6 fractions, prior to busulfan, 12 mg/kg (n = 4) or 9 mg/kg (n = 5), and cyclophosphamide 120 mg/kg. Three patients who had previously undergone radiation therapy received busulfan (14 mg/kg) and cyclophosphamide (120 mg/kg). This modified total body irradiation regimen was performed using a linear accelerator, in 1.5 Gy fractions, with lung and liver

Table 3.2-1 Characteristics and outcome of patients with multiple myeloma after allogeneic stem cell transplantation.

Patient	Sex	Age	Stage	Pre-transplant regimens	Status at transplant	Conditioning regimen	Time from Dx to transplant (months)	Response to transplant	Response to DLI	Follow-up (months)
1	F	47	IIIA	7x MP/5xVAD	2.PR	TMI/BU/CY	16	CR	–	CR 27+
2	M	42	IIA	6xVAD	1.PR	TMI/BU/CY	12	PR	CR	CR 43+
3	F	47	IIA	18xMP	3.PR	TMI/BU/CY	58	–	–	Died: organ-failure day 13
4	F	42	IIIA	4xMP/3xVAD	2.PR	BU/CY	13	PR	None	Alive with disease: 61+
5	M	45	IIIA	4xVAD	1.PR	TMI/BU/CY	8	PR	PR	DLI after PD:Alive in PR 50+
6	M	53	IIA	14xVCAP	2.PR	TMI/BU/CY	24	CR	–	CR 18+
7	M	49	IIIA	7xVCAP / 1xMP	1.PR	BU/CY	10	PR	CR	CR after DLI: CR 18+
8	M	41	IIIB	4xVAD / 2xCyclo	1.PR	TMI/BU/CY	12	CR	–	CR 60+
9	M	42	IIA	4xID	1.PR	TMI/BU/CY	6	PR	–	PR 22+
10	M	29	IIIA	4xVAD	m.R.	TMI/BU/CY	8	PR	–	PD, alive 27+
11	M	50	IIA	4xID	1.PR	TMI/BU/CY	12	–	–	Died GvHD day 43
12	M	43	IIA	4xID	1.PR	BU/CY	14	CR	–	CR 5+

shielding. After radiation, electron beams were given to shielded rib areas [21]. Busulfan was administered orally in 4 separate doses, daily, for 3.5 days (days –8 to –5); cyclophosphamide (60 mg/kg) was infused (1 h) on consecutive days (days –3 and –2). To prevent busulfan-induced seizures, phenytoin was given, ending 2 days after busulfan-therapy. Uroepithelial prophylaxis was achieved with hyperhydration and mesna. Bone marrow or peripheral blood stem cells were infused 24–48 h after the last cyclophosphamide administration (day 0). The stem cell source was bone marrow in 10 patients, and peripheral blood stem cells in 2 patients. Regimen-related toxicity was graded using the Bearman score [22]. The maximum score for each organ system was recorded. Attempts were made to separate toxicities due to GvHD from treatment-related toxicity. Veno-occlusive disease of the liver was graded according to the Seattle criteria [16].

GvHD prophylaxis

Rabbit anti-thymocyte globulin (Fresenius, Bad Homburg, Germany) was given to all patients as part of the preparative regimen. Eleven patients received a dose of 30 mg/kg over 12 hours on days –3, –2 and –1, and 1 patient received a dose of ATG of 30 mg/kg on day –3. Further GvHD prophylaxis consisted of cyclosporine A, 3 mg/kg, given from day –1 to six months post transplantation. Cyclosporin A, adjusted to therapeutic dose level, was tapered from day 84 and discontinued at day 180. Methotrexate (10 mg/m²) was given on days 1, 3 and 6 post transplantation. Standard criteria were used for acute and chronic GvHD [17].

Definition of response

Complete response (CR) was defined as follows: 95% plasma cells with normal morphology in bone marrow aspirate, absence of monoclonal protein on serum electrophoresis and immunofixation, and, if present, no detectable Bence-Jones protein (BJP) in a 24-hour urine specimen. A partial response (PR) was defined as decrease of at least 50% of serum paraprotein level or of BJP concentration in urine. Patients with reduced PR were defined as minor responders (mR). An increase in paraprotein concentration > 25% was termed progressive disease, whereas relapse was defined as paraprotein reappearance and/or marrow infiltration.

Results

Engraftment

No graft failure was observed. The median time elapsed to reach a WBC count of $1.0 \times 10^9/l$ was 16 days (range 11–5). Platelet count > $20 \times 10^9/l$, and independence from platelet transfusion, was reached at a median of 26 days (range 16–52).

GvHD

Three patients developed grade I acute GvHD, and grade II–IV acute GvHD occurred in 3 patients (27%). Severe grade III and IV GvHD was seen in only 1 patient, who died from acute GvHD. Chronic GvHD was evaluated in

10 patients who survived day 80 post BMT. The incidence of chronic GvHD was but 20%, mostly with limited disease. However, two patients who received DLI to intensify tumour regression developed acute GvHD grade II and III, respectively, with one, experiencing extensive GvHD, requiring further immunosuppression by means of prednisone or cyclosporine A.

Treatment-related toxicity

The major toxicity was mucositis. Grade II toxicity, according to the Bearman score, was noted in 10 patients, whereas 2 patients experienced grade III toxicity, requiring prophylactic intubation. Both patients were treated with TMI, cyclophosphamide and busulfan, 12 and 9 mg/kg, respectively. Liver toxicity grade II was seen in 6 patients, grade I in 2 patients, while 4 patients remained free of liver toxicity. One patient developed EBV-associated lymphoma, which resolved completely after anti-CD20 therapy and T-cell infusion. One patient died of severe GvHD grade IV and one developed multiorgan failure on day +13, resulting in a treatment-related mortality of 17%.

Response to BMT

A complete response after allogeneic transplantation was seen in 4 patients (40%), while 6 patients were in partial remission. Two of the patients with partial remission received donor lymphocytes 8 and 14 months after stem cell transplantation, to induce further tumour reduction; they subsequently converted to complete remission, thus increasing the rate of complete remission to 60%.

Overall and progression-free survival

After a median follow-up of 25 months (range 5–62), the estimated overall survival at three years for all patients is 83 per cent (CI 95%: 68%–98%). The estimated progression-free survival at three years is 61 per cent (CI 95%:

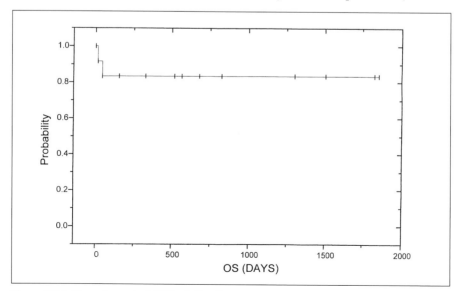

Figure 3.2-1 Overall survival (OS) of all patients.

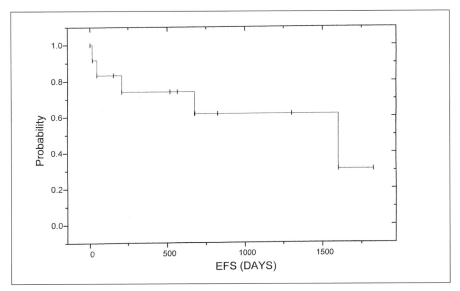

Figure 3.2-2 Event-free survival (EFS) of all patients.

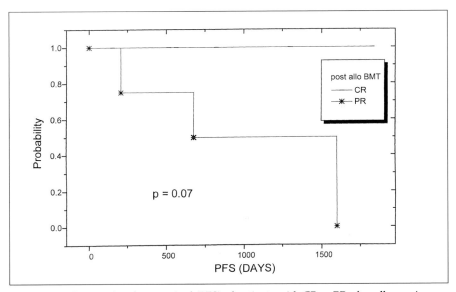

Figure 3.2-3 Progression-free survival (PFS) of patients with CR or PR after allogeneic transplantation.

32%–90%). The Kaplan-Meier survival curves for overall and event-free survival are shown in Figure 3.2-1 and Figure 3.2-2. No patient with CR after allogeneic transplantation relapsed during the follow-up, while 3 out of 6 patients, with only PR after transplantation, progressed within 3 years (p = 0.07) (Fig. 3.2-3). Two patients with PR after allogeneic transplantation (positive immunofixation) received donor lymphocyte infusions (1.5 x 10^8 and 1 x 10^7 CD3+ cells/kg) 8 and 14 months after transplantation, respectively. Both patients developed acute (grade II or III) and chronic GvHD, which resolved after steroid and cyclosporine treatment. Both patients converted from PR to CR after 3 and 4 months, respectively. Two patients with relapse received donor lymphocyte infusion (3 x 10^7 CD3+ cells/kg). One patient did not respond, the second patient experienced a second PR with limited chronic GvHD.

Discussion

Allogeneic stem cell transplantation is probably the most promising approach to the treatment of patients with multiple myeloma. Despite the higher rate of complete remissions and a lower rate of relapse in comparison to autologous transplantation, the treatment-related mortality of 35–57% reported by the EBMT [44], by the Société Française [15] and by the Seattle group [3], allogeneic stem cell transplantation in multiple myeloma remains highly controversial. The severe initial therapy, or the patients refractory to treatment, as well as the development of severe graft-versus-host disease are mainly responsible for the high score in treatment-related mortality. This explains why studies involving an earlier onset for transplantation, PBSC as stem cell source, T-cell depletion to prevent GvHD achieved a lower figure of about 20% in treatment-related mortality [14,19]. A recent analysis of the EBMT also reported a lower transplant-related mortality (20%) with patients transplanted after 1995 as compared to patients who underwent transplantation before 1995 (40%) [9]. Because of the proven graft-versus-myeloma effect [20,21], T-cell depletion reduced GvHD, but suffered from higher relapse rates [19]. Our group and others [7,10,11,22] showed that anti-thymocyte globulin (ATG), as part of the conditioning regimen, resulted in a low incidence of severe GvHD, without apparent increase in relapses in unrelated stem cell transplantation. The first and foremost objective of our study therefore was to lower TRM by avoiding severe GvHD. We incorporated ATG in the preparative regimen of either modified total body irradiation, busulfan and cyclophosphamide or busulfan and cyclo-phosphamide. ATG is a rabbit-anti-human immunoglobulin. After immuniza-tion, using cells from a T-lymphoblast cell line (Jurkat T-cell line), these highly purified specific antibodies are directed against lymphoblastic T-cells, and thus induce *in vivo* T-cell depletion via opsonization and lysis, following complement activation. Pharmacokinetic studies performed with ATG using ELISA techniques and an inhibitory effect on phytohaemagglutinin-induced blasto-genesis showed a dose-dependent effect. Rabbit IgG was still detectable at least four weeks after administration, and the effect of the phytohaemagglutinin response on normal mononuclear cells lasted up to four days post trans-plantation [5]. Therefore, the effect of ATG as part of the pretransplant con-ditioning regimen is likely to be an *in vivo* T-cell effect on the bone marrow of the donor.

The incidence of grade II–IV acute GvHD in our study was only 27%, but one patient developed severe and fatal acute grade IV GvHD. The incidence of chronic GvHD was similarly low, only 20%. The toxicity of the conditioning regimen was mainly stomatitis of grade II at least in all patients. Two patients experienced grade III toxicity, requiring mechanical ventilation. Both patients died, one of multi-organ failure, the other of severe GvHD, resulting in a treatment-related mortality of 17%.

The second aim of our study was to achieve a high rate of complete remission, known to be associated with long-term disease-free survival [3,4]. The modified total body irradiation with lung and liver shielding (total marrow irradiation) in combination with busulfan and cyclophosphamide was chosen after a high percentage of complete response was observed in a phase II trial followed by autologous transplantation [6]. Forty per cent of the patients achieved complete remission after allogeneic transplantation, while the remaining patients went into partial remission. Two of the patients with partial remission received donor lymphocyte infusions for further tumour reduction and converted to continuous complete remission 12 and 28 months after DLI [12], which increased the rate of complete remission to 60%. No patient with CR, but 3 out of 4 patients with PR suffered tumour progression during follow-up, demonstrating the necessity of further tumour reduction by donor lymphocytes in patients with incomplete remission after allogeneic stem cell transplantation. DLI-toxicity, however, caused considerable acute and chronic GvHD, which is why further studies, in order to optimize the T-cell dose, are imperative.

The proven graft-versus-myeloma effect of allogeneic T-cells and the introduction of less toxic non-myeloablative conditioning regimens for allogeneic transplantation should offer new therapeutic approaches towards a better treatment of multiple myeloma.

We conclude that the conditioning regimen with modified TBI, busulfan and cyclophosphamide is able to induce a high CR rate after allogeneic stem cell transplantation, and that DLI should be administered to patients with incomplete response after transplantation. The incorporation of anti-thymocyte globulin may prevent severe GvHD without apparent increase in relapse.

Acknowledgements

We thank the staff of the BMT unit for providing excellent care for our patients, and the medical technicians for their excellent work in the BMT laboratory.

References

1. ANDERSON, K.C., *et al.*: Monoclonal antibody purged bone marrow transplantation therapy for multiple myeloma. Blood 82 (1993) 2568–2576.
2. BEARMAN, S.I., *et al.*: Regimen-related toxicity in patients undergoing bone marrow transplantation. J Clin Oncol 6 (1988) 1562–1568.
3. BENSINGER, W., *et al.*: Allogeneic marrow transplantation for multiple myeloma: an analysis of risk factors on outcome. Blood 88 (1996) 2787–2793.
4. BJÖRKSTRAND, B., *et al.*: Allogeneic bone marrow transplantation vs autologous stem cell transplantation in multiple myeloma: a retrospective case-matched study from the European Group for Blood and Marrow Transplantation. Blood 88 (1996) 4711–4718.
5. EIERMANN, TH., *et al.*: Monitoring anti-thymocyte globulin (ATG) in bone marrow recipients. Bone Marrow Transplantation 23 (1999) 779–781.
6. EINSELE, H., *et al.*: Total marrow irradiation (TMI), busulfan and cyclophosphamide followed by PBSCT in patients with multiple myeloma. Blood 92 (Suppl 1) (1998) 516.

7. FINKE, J., *et al.*: Allogeneic transplantation from unrelated donors: improved outcome using in vivo T-cell depletion. Blood 90 (Suppl 1) (1997) 451.

8. GAHRTON, G., *et al.*: Prognostic factors in allogenic bone marrow transplantation for multiple myeloma. J Clin Oncol 13 (1995) 1312–1322.

9. GAHRTON, G., *et al.*: Progress in allogeneic hematopoietic stem cell transplantation for multiple myeloma. Bone Marrow Transplant 25 (Suppl 1) (2000) 140.

10. KOLB, H.J., *et al.*: Conditioning treatment with Antithymocyte Globulin (ATG) modifies Graft-vs-Host Disease in recipients of marrow from unrelated donors. Blood 86 (Suppl 1) (1995) 952a

11. KRÖGER, N., *et al.*: Anti-Thymocyte-Globulin as part of the preparative regimen prevents acute and chronic Graft-versus-Host disease (GvHD) in allogeneic stem cell transplantation from unrelated donors. Annals of Hematology (2001) 80: 209–215.

12. KRÖGER, N., *et al.*: Donor lymphocyte infusion enhances remission status in patients with persistent disease after allografting for multiple myeloma. British Journal of Haematology 112 (2001) 421–423.

13. LOKHORST, H.M., *et al.*: Donor leukocyte infusions are effective in relapsed multiple myeloma after allogeneic bone marrow transplantation. Blood 90 (10) (1997) 4206–4211.

14. MAJOLINO, I., *et al.*: Allogeneic transplantation of unmanipulated peripheral blood stem cells in patients with multiple myeloma. Bone Marrow Transplant 22 (1998) 449–455.

15. MARIT, G., *et al.*: Allogeneic stem cell transplantation in multiple myeloma: a report of the Société Française de Greffe de Moelle. Blood 10 (Suppl 1) (1997) 996.

16. MCDONALD, G.B., *et al.*: Veno-occlusive disease of the liver and multiorgan failure after bone marrow transplantation: a cohort study of 355 patients. Ann Intern Med 118 (1993) 255–267.

17. PRZEPIORKA, K.M., *et al.*: 1994 Consensus Conference on acute GvHD-grading. Bone Marrow Transplantat 15 (1995) 825–828.

18. REECE, D.E., *et al.*: Treatment of myeloma using intensive therapy and allogeneic bone marrow transplantation. Bone Marrow Transplant 15 (1995) 117–123.

19. SCHLOSSMAN, R.L., *et al.*: Similar disease-free survival after allografting and autografting for multiple myeloma. Blood 10 (Suppl 1) (1997) 994 .

20. TRICOT, G., *et al.*: Graft-versus-myeloma effect: proof of a principle. Blood 87 (1996) 1196–1198.

21. VERDONCK, L., *et al.*: Graft-versus-myeloma effect in two cases. Lancet 347 (1996) 800–801.

22. ZANDER, A.R., *et al.*: Use of a five-agent GvHD prevention regimen in recipients of unrelated donor marrow. Bone Marrow Transplantation 23 (1999) 889–893.

3.3 Remission of Severe Steroid-Refractory Acute GvHD Following Allogeneic PBSCT Can Be Induced by the IL-2R-Antagonist Basiliximab

Knauf, W. U.*, I. W. Blau, T. Fietz, H. Schrezenmeier, E. Thiel

Bone Marrow Transplantation Unit, Medizinische Klinik III, Universitätsklinik Benjamin Franklin, Freie Universität Berlin, Berlin, Germany

* To whom correspondence should be addressed (wolfgang.knauf@medizin.fu-berlin.de)

Summary

Activated T-cells which express the α-chain (CD25) of the interleukin-2 receptor complex (IL-2R) are involved in the development of graft-versus-host disease (GvHD) after allogeneic haematopoietic stem cell transplantation. Therefore, monoclonal antibodies against CD25 seem to be an attractive option to keep graft-versus-host disease under control. To further test this hypothesis, we initiated a pilot study on feasibility and efficacy of basiliximab, an IL-2R antagonist, which is currently used to prevent and treat graft rejection after solid organ transplantation. Six patients (4 with AML, 1 with ALL/Ph1+, 1 with CML/CP1) entered the trial. Two patients received an HLA-identical sibling graft, while the others had a matched unrelated donor (n = 3) or a mismatched unrelated donor (n = 1). GvHD prophylaxis consisted of CSA (n = 2), CSA+MMF (n = 2), CSA+MMF+ATG (n = 1), and CSA+MTX (n = 1), respectively. Nonetheless, all the six patients developed acute skin and/or intestinal GvHD, which was progressive despite the i.v. administration of daily 1–2 mg/kg body weight steroids plus i.v. CSA. After 20 mg basiliximab had been additionally given on day 0 and day 4, clinical signs of GvHD disappeared completely or were grade I within one week in four patients. In another patient skin GvHD regressed from grade IV to grade I while intestinal GvHD grade IV remained unchanged. The remaining patient had refractory GvHD. These latter two patients ultimately succumbed to GvHD. Interestingly, two patients experienced recurrence of GvHD while tapering steroids. In both cases retreatment with basiliximab led to complete remission of GvHD. Taken together, encouraging results have been achieved with the IL-2R antagonist basiliximab in the treatment of severe steroid-refractory GvHD. However, more patients and a longer follow-up are needed to evaluate this antibody-based therapy of GvHD.

Introduction

Acute graft-versus-host disease (aGvHD) remains a major cause of morbidity and mortality after allogeneic transplantation of haematopoietic stem cells, despite sophisticated DNA typing methods and various regimens used for GvHD prophylaxis. Triggered by tissue damage due to the conditioning treatment or as a result of infectious challenge, a cascade of cytokine-driven cell activation steps is initiated which leads to deleterious local inflammation in target organs such as skin, liver, and gut [2]. A predominant role within this cascade is shared by activated T-cells which are characterized by the expression of the α-chain of the IL-2 receptor complex (IL-2R). This α-chain (CD25) confers high-affinity properties on the IL-2R heteromultimer additionally built by the β-chain (CD122) and the γ-chain, respectively [5]. Interaction of IL-2R with its ligand IL-2 triggers activation of the ras pathway and results in lymphocyte proliferation and differentiation [5]. Therefore, selective blockage of the IL-2Rα could be an attractive way to inhibit activation of alloreactive T-cells and to discontinue the cascade leading to GvHD.

Basiliximab is a monoclonal chimeric human-mouse antibody consisting of variable regions of the mouse antiCD25 antibody RFT5 and the constant regions of the human IgG1 heavy and κ light chains. The RFT5 part of basiliximab binds with high affinity to CD25, while the human IgG1 part significantly reduces the risk of induction of human anti-mouse antibodies (*Novartis*, data on file).

This prompted us to test the efficacy and tolerability of basiliximab in an unselected series of patients suffering from severe steroid-refractory aGvHD following allografting with peripheral, blood-derived haematopoietic stem cells.

Patients and methods

Between May 2000 and April 2001, a cohort of six consecutive patients suffering from severe steroid-refractory aGvHD were enrolled into the trial. All these patients had been transplanted with an allogeneic peripheral, blood-derived haematopoietic stem cell graft. Indication for transplantation was AML in four patients, Philadelphia-chromosome positive ALL in one patient, and CML in first chronic phase in one patient, respectively. Except for the patient with CML, all other patients were transplanted in first haematological remission. Median age of the three women and three men was 42 years (range 30–54 years). Conditioning therapy consisted of hyperfractionated TBI (12 Gy) plus cyclophosphamide 120 mg/kg body weight (BW) in five patients, and of treosulfan 30 mg/kg (BW) plus fludarabine 25 mg/sqm in one patient. According to currently activated protocols, GvHD prophylaxis consisted of cyclosporine alone in two patients, cyclosporine plus MMF (mycophenolate mofetil) in two patients, cyclosporine plus MMF plus ATG in one patient, and cyclosporine plus MTX in one patient, respectively. No haematopoietic growth factors were administered after transplantation.

Grading of aGvHD followed the guidelines of the 1994 consensus conference [6]. In case aGvHD developed, steroids 1–2 mg/kg BW/daily were added to the underlying immunosuppressive treatment. Whenever GvHD was found to be progressive or showed clinically no amelioration within 48 hours, the patient was eligible to enter the trial.

Anti-CD25 monoclonal antibody basiliximab (Novartis, Basle, CH) was given i.v. at a fixed cumulative dose of 40 mg, split into two doses of 20 mg each on days 0 and 4, while the formerly given immunosuppression continued. GvHD was evaluated daily, and best response was documented.

Complete remission of GvHD was diagnosed whenever clinical signs of

GvHD completely disappeared. Partial remission was defined in case of downgrading by at least one unit in one target organ. Clinical characteristics of the patients are summarized in Table 3.3-1.

Table 3.3-1 Patient characteristics.

Age	Diagnosis (number)	HLA match		GvHD prophylaxis	
42 years	AML (4)	ident. sib.	(2)	CSA	(2)
(median)	CML (1)	MUD	(3)	CSA + MTX	(1)
	ALL (1)	MMUD	(1)	CSA + MMF	(2)
				CSA + MMF + ATG	(1)

AML = acute myeloid leukaemia, CML = chronic myelogenous leukaemia, ALL = acute lymphoblastic leukaemia, ident. sib. = identical sibling, MUD = matched unrelated donor, MMUD = mismatched unrelated donor, CSA = cyclosporine A, MTX = methotrexate, MMF = mycophenolat mofetil, ATG = anti-thymocyte globulin

Results

Clinical signs of GvHD disappeared completely in three patients within one week, while two other patients attained PR: One patient with grade I GvHD of the skin (former grade III), and also grade I GvHD of the skin in another patient who, in addition, experienced refractory grade IV GvHD of the gut. One patient showed no signs of response. The latter two patients ultimately succumbed to GvHD.

Interestingly, GvHD reappeared in two patients while tapering down steroids. These patients were treated again with basiliximab and reached stable CR. In another patient, AML relapsed at day 90 post transplant, accompanied by cutaneous grade I GvHD. No anti-GvHD treatment was initiated. This particular patient had stable GvHD and smouldering leukaemia with 10% residual donor haematopoiesis as shown by sex chromosome FISH (last follow-up was on day 120).

No side effects attributable to basiliximab were noted. A summary of the results is listed in Table 3.3-2.

Table 3.3-2 Effects of basiliximab on GvHD.

Patients	GvHD grade prior to anti-IL-2R	GvHD grade post anti-IL-2R
AML	(skin) III	I
AML	(skin) III	0
AML	(skin) III	0
AML	(skin) IV	I
	(gut) IV	IV
CML	(gut) III	0
ALL	(skin) III	II
	(gut) III	III

Grading of GvHD followed the guidelines of the 1994 consensus conference [6].

Discussion

Steroid-refractory GvHD is a serious complication in the aftermath of allogeneic haematological stem cell transplantation and contributes significantly to the transplant-related mortality. Moreover, besides the diabetogenic effect, steroids favour fluid retention in patients who already may suffer from capillary leak syndrome due to the "cytokine storm". Therefore, long-term therapy with high doses of steroids should be avoided. Owing to this complexity, a treatment targeted towards the GvHD-promoting CD25+-cells offers an attractive alternative.

With the use of murine monoclonal antibodies against CD25, which represents the IL-2-receptor α-chain, complete response rates in the range of 10%–88% have been reported [1,3,8]. However, murine antibodies are rather immunogenic when administered to man. The human-mouse chimeric monoclonal antibody basiliximab is characterized by a high binding affinity which encourages low-dose treatment, and was found to induce a very low rate of immunization [4]. It has been approved for renal graft rejection in the USA and the European Community. In our present study, it was found to be effective in inducing remission of severe steroid-refractory GvHD following allogeneic PBSCT.

Remissions became clinically apparent within 48–72 hours after initiation of therapy. In analogy to the procedure used in renal allografted patients, a second dose of basiliximab was administered on day 4. Shortly thereafter, GvHD had completely resolved in three patients. No side effects attributable to immunization were noted after the second antibody infusion. The optimal duration of therapy with basiliximab is unclear, as is its efficacy in case of GvHD recurrence. We saw two patients experiencing recurrence of GvHD after an initially successful treatment, while remission remained stable in three other cases. Incomplete donor/recipient chimerism, infections, or ongoing tissue damage may contribute to an upregulation of CD25 on T-cells, monocytes, and NK-cells, leading to GvHD whenever plasma levels of basiliximab decrease below a critical threshold. However, both patients achieved stable complete remission of GvHD shortly after a second course of basiliximab on day 0 and, in addition, on day 4.

The treatment of GvHD, using monoclonal antibodies, has also been treated in other reports [7]. Daclizumab, the IL-2R-antibody used in one particular study, induced remissions in 29% – 47% of the patients, relative to the dosage given. Due to its lower receptor affinity, daclizumab has to be administered repetitively with a higher cumulative dosage than basiliximab. This could be a disadvantage with regard to the risk of immunization as well as to cost effectiveness.

Considering the reduced number of patients, and, therefore, the limited experience gained from the clinical course of this small cohort, we feel that basiliximab is an effective agent to be used against severe aGvHD following allogeneic PBSCT. The fact that responses occur rapidly should be of assistance when deciding whether or not a change in the therapeutic strategy has to be envisaged without too great a loss of time. In our opinion, these preliminary observations make basiliximab an attractive therapeutic option for the successful treatment of aGvHD.

References

1. CUTHBERT, R.J.G., *et al.*: Anti-interleukin-2 receptor monoclonal antibody (BT563) in the treatment of severe acute GVHD refractory to systemic corticosteroid therapy. Bone Marrow Transpl 10 (1991) 451.
2. FERRARA, J.L.M., J.H. ANTIN: The pathophysiology of graft-versus-host disease. In: E. D. Thomas, K. G. Blume, S.J. Forman (eds.) Hematopoietic Cell Transplantation, 2nd edition, Blackwell Science (1999) 305.
3. HERBELIN, C., *et al.*: Treatment of steroid resistant acute graft-versus-host disease with an anti-IL-2-receptor monoclonal antibody (BT563) in children who received T-cell-depleted, partially matched, related bone marrow transplants. Bone Marrow Transpl 13 (1994) 563.
4. KOVARIK, J., *et al.*: Prolonged immunosuppressive effect and minimal immunogenicity from chimeric (CD25) monoclonal antibody SDZ CHI 621 in renal transplantation. Transpl Proc 28 (1996) 913.
5. NELSON, B.H., D.M. WILLERFORD: Biology of the interleukin-2-receptor. Adv Immunol 70 (1998) 1.
6. PRZEPIORKA, D., *et al.*: Report of the 1994 consensus conference on acute GvHD grading. Bone Marrow Transpl 15 (1995) 825.
7. PRZEPIORKA, D., *et al.*: Daclizumab, a humanized anti-interleukin-2 receptor alpha chain antibody, for the treatment of acute graft-versus-host disease. Blood 95 (2000) 83.
8. TILEY, C., *et al.*: Treatment of acute graft-versus-host disease with a murine monoclonal antibody to the IL-2 receptor. Bone Marrow Transpl 7 (1991) 151.

Part Four
Miscellaneous / Short Communications*

4.1 Clinical Outcome of Cord Blood Transplantation. A Summary of the Tokyo Cord Blood Bank (as integral part of the *Japan Cord Blood Bank Network*)

Takahashi T. A., T. Nagamura-Inoue, H. Nagayama, S. Asano

Division of Cell Processing, The Institute of Medical Science, The University of Tokyo, Shirokanedai 4-6-1, Minato-ku, Tokyo, Japan

Summary

Since the Tokyo Cord Blood Bank started cryopreserving cord blood, more than 2,500 units have been collected and 780 units registered with the *Japan Cord Blood Bank Network*. Now in Japan, doctors, patients and the patient's family may search for and find the suitable cord blood for the recipient. Nationwide, 4,500 units are now registered in this *Network*, and more than 334 cord blood transplants were performed from 1997 to December 2000. By December 2000, the Tokyo Cord Blood Bank had provided 63 units for recipients in Japan, the United States and New Zealand. In 1998, we performed the first successful cord blood transplantation of an HLA2/6 loci-mismatched sample in an adult recipient. Since then, twenty-two adult patients, aged from 15 to 50 years, have received cord blood transplants (CBT) with a dose of more than 1.6×10^7/kg body weight of all nucleated cells (ANCs) from Tokyo Cord Blood Bank. The incidence of myeloid engraftment in adults and children was 11/15 (73%) and 18/25 (72%), respectively. In 11 adult recipients who had engraftment, neutrophil and platelet recovery was not delayed as compared to children. Overall survival of adult patients demonstrated no significant difference to paediatric patients. These clinical outcomes suggest that cord blood, using at least 2×10^7/kg nucleated cells, can be an acceptable source of haematopoietic stem cells, even for adult recipients.

Introduction

Unrelated allogeneic bone marrow transplantation can cure haematopoietic disorders including leukaemia, lymphoma, immunodeficiency syndrome and some metabolic disorders. Its success, however, depends on how rapidly identification of HLA-identical donors can be achieved, how fast the transplantation can be performed, and how good acute GvHD can be controlled. Unrelated umbilical cord blood transplantation has been overcoming these problems, although other problems remain to be solved. Over the past six years, more than 600 cases of placental and umbilical cord blood transplantation from unrelated donors have been reported, suggesting abundant resources for haematopoietic stem cells. RUBINSTEIN *et al.* reported that myeloid engraftment correlated significantly with recipient age, the number of ANCs per kg weight in the graft, the type of disease, the extent of HLA disparity and the transplantation centre, although age was not independently predictive in multivariate analysis [1,2,4,5]. In previous papers, elderly patients were at disadvantage because of their body weight, which precluded receiving an appropriate dose of nucleated cells. However, in the absence of HLA-identical or HLA-compatible (up to two loci mismatched) bone marrow donors, adult recipients may be in urgent need of cord blood. In this case, assessing the disadvantage of CBT is imperative.

In this report, we summarize the clinical results obtained in 44 registered patients, including 18 adult patients who received CBT, supplied by our blood bank, from 1997 to December 2000.

Materials and methods

Harvesting of placental and umbilical blood and collection of data on donors

Placental umbilical cord blood was collected from freshly delivered placenta at Hamada Hospital, Yamaguchi Hospital, San-ikukai Hospital, Bokutoh Hospital, Gynaecology Units of Keio University School of Medicine, and Juntendoh University School of Medicine, Urayasu Hospital. Trained staff members harvested blood from placenta and umbilical cord, and collected blood specimens from each mother. Written informed consent was also obtained, as were abstracts of interviews including data on family history and the medical records of mothers and children. The procedure was approved by the institutional review board of the Institute of Medical Science from Tokyo University.

Processing and cryopreservation

The processing and cryopreservation methods were performed as described previously, with some modifications [6]. Briefly: before centrifugation, hydroxyethyl starch (HES) was added to CPD-cord blood up to a final concentration of 1.2%. The leukocyte-enriched supernatant was separated, and the collected cells were sedimented by centrifugation. The sedimented WBC were resuspended in supernatant plasma, and dimethyl sulphoxide (DMSO) plus dextran-40 added up to a final concentration of 10% (vol/vol) DMSO. Cryopreservation was performed according to the protocol of the New York Blood Center [6]. Aliquots were cryopreserved by programmed freezing in a BioArchive liquid nitrogen tank.

Removal of hypertonic cryoprotectant

DMSO was removed to less than 5% of the total volume [6], after thawing cord blood in a water bath at 37° C, diluted with an equal volume of a solution containing 2.5% human albumin (Japan Red Cross) and 5% dextran-40 (Baxter) in isotonic saline, and then centrifuged. The supernatant was removed, and albumin and dextran added to a final volume of about 70 ml. Prior to injection, the processed cells were brought to 37°C.

Patients

For the purpose of CBT, the standard acceptable dose of ANCs was tentatively set at a value $> 2 \times 10^7$/kg BW, and, as outlined by the Japan Cord Blood Bank

Network, the standard for an acceptable HLA match was defined as a match of 4/6 loci.

Fifty-five patients were transplanted with cord blood in 28 different transplant centres, including one US centre; we analysed only the 44 patients registered at the Tokyo Cord Blood Bank data centre.

Statistical analysis

The probability of event-free survival was calculated by Kaplan-Meier analysis drawn in Jump (SAS Institute). Data on adverse events, i.e. death, graft failure, relapse, or death from other causes were censored.

Results and discussion

Patients characteristics

Due to the volume limitation encountered in harvested cord blood, and, thus, the limited number of nucleated cells, CBT would appear to be particularly suitable for transplant purposes in children. We nevertheless endeavoured to also save adult patients lacking suitable bone marrow donors, and urgently needing cord blood as a stem cell source. Although the disease background in children and adults was quite different, we proceeded as summarized in Table 4.1-1, thereby trying to resolve the problem of CBT in adults.

Twenty-six patients were children < 14 years, 18 were adults > 15 years, the median age being 4.9 ± 4.1 yrs and 30.5 ± 11.7 yrs, respectively. Body weight

Table 4.1-1 Demographic and clinical characteristics of 56 patients who received cord blood from Tokyo CB bank (II).

No. of patients		Children (< 15 years)	Adults (≥ 15 years)
		26	18
Age		4.9 ± 4.1	30.5 ± 11.5
		(range 0.5–10)	*(range 15–50)*
Disease	Acute leukaemia		
	ALL	12	1
	AML	6	8
	AMixL	0	1
	Lymphoma	0	4
	MDS	0	4
	Neuroblastoma	1	0
	Aplastic anaemia	1	0
	Immunodeficiency	1	0
	Other	Duncan's syndrome = 1	0
		Ohmmen's syndrome = 2	
		EB-related HP = 2	
Nucleated cell dose (x 10^7/kg/BW)		5.6 ± 3.4	2.7 ± 0.7
		(range 1.8–16.3)	*(range 1.63–4.23)*
HLA match	3	1	2
	4	12	7
	5	12	8
	6	1	1

median was 18.8 ± 13.3 kg in children, and 51.5 ± 9.7 kg in adults. With respect to BW, the transplanted cell dose (ANCs at cryopreservation) was 5.6 ± 3.5 x 10^7 cells/kg (range: 1.77–16.3 x 10^7/kg) in children, in adults, however, only half the dose with 2.7 ± 0.7 x 10^7 cells/kg (range: 1.63–4.23 x 10^7/kg).

The underlying diseases in children were: acute lymphocytic leukaemia (ALL) (n = 12), acute myelogenous leukaemia (AML) (n = 6), aplastic anaemia (n = 1), neuroblastoma (n = 1), severe combined immunodeficiency disease (SCID) (n = 1), Ohmmen's syndrome (n = 2), Duncan's syndrome (n = 1), other (n = 2); and in adults: haematopoietic malignancies including ALL (n = 1), AML, AMixL (n = 1), lymphoma (n = 4), myelodysplastic syndrome (MDS) (n = 4).

Thirteen adult patients were transplanted as described, whereas 5 patients received transplants without diluted DMSO in the supernatant. Only four of the twenty-six child recipients received transplants in which DMSO had been removed.

Engraftment

In elderly patients, and because of their body weight, delayed engraftment may represent a major problem. Out of 25 child patients (except for one who died on day 16), 18 (72%) patients engrafted, one patient showed mixed recovery and 6 failed to engraft. In fifteen adult patients, except for 3 who died within 4 weeks after CBT without evaluation of engraftment, 11 (73%) patients engrafted, one showed mixed recovery, and engraftment failed in 3 patients. The highest incidence of graft failure occurred in the age group from 2 to 5, with graft failure in 5 out of 9 patients (56%), including 3 ALL, 1 AML and 1 Duncan's syndrome; 1 showed mixed recovery. In the patients who obtained

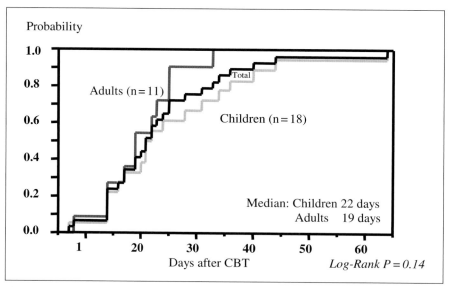

Figure 4.1-1 Probability of achieving PLT > 20 x 10^9/L after CBT between children and adults.

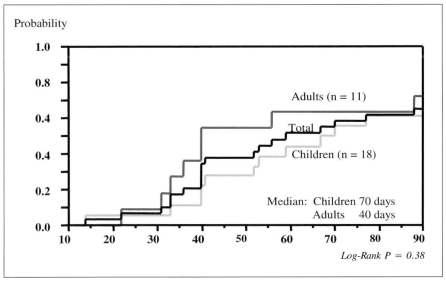

Figure 4.1-2 Probability of achieving PLT > 20 x 10⁹/L after CBT between adults and children.

myeloid engraftment, neutrophil recovery with more than 0.5×10^9/L occurred at a median 22 days in child patients (n = 18) and of 19 days in adult patients (n = 11) (Fig. 4.1-1). Platelet recovery of more than 20×10^9/L was achieved at a median 70 days in child patients and 40 days in adult patients (Fig. 4.1-2), although not statistically significant (p = 0.33).

Our preliminary results suggest that haematopoietic recovery from cord blood showed no difference in adults as compared to child patients, especially considering the recovery rate of neutrophils in the group which successfully engrafted, although platelet recovery rate and incidence have yet to be resolved. Comparing the myeloid recovery rate, one should be careful with respect to the background. In adults, nine patients received grafts using the DMSO removal procedure, while only one child patient received a similar graft. In the future, it will be necessary to evaluate the effects on the recovery rate in the same population.

Acute GvHD

Acute graft-versus-host disease (GvHD) is one of the main causes of unrelated bone marrow transplantation (UBMT), however, acute GvHD in CBT has been known to be mild and less severe than those of UBMT. As previously reported, no patients died of acute GvHD in this study. The incidence of GvHD was as follows: Of the 18 child patients with myeloid engraftment, grade 0 GvHD occurred in 5, grade I in 5, grade II in 5, and grade III in 3; grade IV was not observed. In the 11 adult patients with engraftment the GvHD figures read as follows: grade 0 = 4, grade I = 5, grade II = 2; Grade III and IV were not seen (Table 4.1-3).

Table 4.1-2 Cumulative incidence of myeloid engraftment among recipients of CBT.

		Children		Adults	
		Subtotal	Engraftment	Subtotal	Engraftment
Overall		25	18 (72%)	15	11 (73%)
Age					
< 2 yrs		7	7 (100%)		
2–5 yrs		9	3 (33%)		
6–11 yrs		7	5 (83%)		
12–14 yrs		2	4 (100%)		
≥ 15 yrs				15	11 (73%)
No. of leukocytes before cryopreservation					
> 2.5 x 10^7/kg		2	2	7	4 (57%)
2.5-4.9 x 10^7/kg		10	9 (90%)	8	7 (88%)
> 5 x 10^7/kg		13	7 (54%)	0	–
Washing before transplant					
Non-wash	25	21	17 (81%)	4	3
Wash	15	4	1	11	8 (73%)
No. of HLA-A, B, and DR (B1) mismatches					
0	2	1	1	1	1
1	17	11	9 (82%)	6	5 (83%)
2	18	12	7 (63%)	6	4 (67%)
3	4	1	1	2	3
Transplant before CBT					
0	30	18	14	11	9
auto	4	2	0	3	1
allo	3	2	0	0	–
auto + allo	3	2	2	1	1

Recipient numbers exclude the patients who died before 30 days with no engraftment observed.

Table 4.1-3 Acute GvHD.

	Children (n = 26)	Adults (n = 18)
Engraftment	18	11
Grade 0	5 (28%)	4 (33%)
Grade I	5 (28%)	5 (45%)
Grade II	5 (28%)	2 (18%)
Grade III	3	0
Grade IV	0	0

Survival

In the overall survival and event-free survival, there was no significant difference between child and adult patients (Fig. 4.1-3). The only obvious effect on the cause of death was the stage of disease at transplantation in all patients with acute leukaemia (Fig. 4.1-4).

Cause of Death

Out of 26 child patients, 14 died and 3 were alive but on relapse. Out of the 14, 8 died of CBT-related cause, including 7 infections and 1 MOF, and the

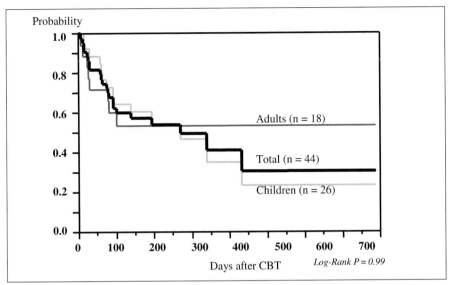

Figure 4.1-3 Probability of overall survival after CBT between adults and children.

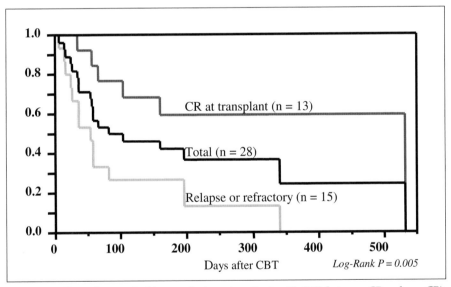

Figure 4.1-4 Event-free survival in acute leukaemia patients with CBT (between CR and non-CR).

remaining 5 died of relapse. One patient died of unknown fever, followed by sudden cardiac arrest. Out of 18 adult patients, 5 died of CBT-related causes, including infection, cardiac toxicity and VOD; the remaining 3 patients died of relapse or tumour progression (see Table 4.1-4).

Conclusion

We conclude that CBT is an acceptable procedure for adult patients if a suitable bone marrow donor is unavailable, and provided a standard level of ANCs can

Table 4.1-4 Clinical outcome of CBT.

	Total (n = 44)	Children (n = 26)	Adults (n = 18)
Alive	22	12	10
On relapse	4	2	2
Event-free	18	10	8
Dead	22	14	8
Transplant-related death	13	8	5
Infection	9	7	2
VOD	2	0	2
MOF	1	1	0
Cardiac toxicity	1	0	1
Unknown	1	1 (Cardiomyositis?)	0
Relapse or progression	8	5	3

be secured from the matching CB Unit. This handicap may be overcome, once the availability of stem cells from CB is resolved, as described in the case reported by PECORA et al. [3]. Finally, a weak acute GvHD may be suspected to also induce a weak graft-versus-leukaemia reaction, eventually leading to relapse. How to prevent relapse after engraftment, however, still remains to be elucidated.

References

1. GLUCKMAN E., et al.: Outcome of cord-blood transplantation from related and unrelated donors. 337 (1997) 373.
2. KURTBERG, J., et al.: Placental blood as a source of haematopoietic stem cells for transplantation into unrelated recipients. The New England J of Medicine 335 (1996) 157.
3. PECORA A.L., et al.: Prompt and durable engraftment in two older adult patients with high-risk chronic myelogenous leukemia (CML) using ex vivo expanded and unmanipulated unrelated umbilical cord blood. Bone Marrow Transplantation 25 (2000) 797.
4. ROCHA, V., et al.: Graft-versus-host disease in children who have received a cord blood or bone marrow transplant from an HLA-identical sibling. The New England J of Medicine 342 (2000) 1846.
5. RUBINSTEIN, P., et al.: Outcomes among 562 recipients of placental-blood transplants from unrelated donors. The New England J of Medicine 339 (1998) 1565.
6. RUBINSTEIN, P., et al.: Processing and cryopreservation of placental/umbilical cord blood for unrelated bone marrow reconstitution. Pro Ntl Acad Sci USA92 (1995) 10119.

4.2 Thalidomide plus CED Chemotherapy as Regimen for Remission Induction in Poor-Prognosis Multiple Myeloma prior to Autologous or Allogeneic Haematopoietic Stem Cell Transplantation

Moehler*, T. M., K. Neben, B. Kasper, L. Kordelas, G. Egerer, M. Görner, A. D. Ho, H. Goldschmidt

University of Heidelberg, Dept. of Haematology/Oncology/Rheumatology, Heidelberg, Germany

*To whom correspondence should be addressed (Thomas_Moehler@med.uni-heidelberg.de)

Summary

Autologous and allogeneic stem cell transplantation (SCT) are currently offered to eligible patients with poor-prognosis multiple myeloma (MM), as part of an intensive treatment regimen to improve progression-free and overall survival. An important prerequisite for the success and durability of transplantation-induced anti-myeloma effects is the induction of the best possible response by induction therapy before SCT. Thalidomide has antiangiogenic effects and was recently shown to have anti-tumour activity in MM.

We report on the safety and efficacy of thalidomide combined with CED chemotherapy (TCED) in 56 patients with poor-prognosis MM (primary refractory, secondary refractory after ABSCT or conventional chemotherapy, plasma cell leukaemia): thalidomide (T) (400 mg p.o. per day, continuously), cyclophosphamide (C) 400 mg/m², etoposide (E) 40 mg/m² both as continuous i.v. infusion d1–4 and dexamethasone (D) 40 mg p.o., repeated after 28 days until best response or for a maximum of 6 cycles. Of 50 patients evaluable for response, 4% (2) achieved CR, 64% (32) PR, 18% (9) MR, 6% (3) stable diseases (SD), 8% (4) PD, resulting in an objective response rate ($\geq$ MR) of 86.6% (intend-to-treat analysis: 76.7%; n = 56). In 1 patient stem cell collection was successfully performed in the G-CSF stimulated period of haematopoietic recovery, following the second cycle of TCED therapy. Subsequent to successful remission induction, 18 patients received autologous (ABSCT; n = 9) or allogeneic stem cell transplantation (n = 9). The estimated median follow-up duration after start of TCED was 14 months. The median progression-free survival was 16 months. The median overall survival time has not been reached so far (12+ months). Severe adverse effects (WHO III/IV) included infectious complications (35.7%) and cardiovascular events (7.1%).

Thalidomide plus CED chemotherapy is an efficient regimen to induce meaningful responses in poor-prognosis MM. For eligible patients with poor-prognosis MM under 65 years, we propose a sequential study design (TCED, autologous SCT, non-myeloablative allogeneic SCT) to achieve long-term remissions.

Introduction

The majority of MM patients suffer from recurrent disease and ultimately succumb to sequelae of this disease [1,10,14,20]. Overall survival of patients with poor-prognosis MM (e.g. primary or secondary resistant disease after conventional chemotherapy and relapse after autologous blood stem cell transplantation) is considered to be between 6 and 12 months. Autologous blood stem cell transplantation has been used in this group of poor-prognosis patients resulting in progression-free and overall survival of 11 and 16 months [22]. The only currently available approach with a chance of long-term remission or even cure in poor-prognosis multiple myeloma is the transplantation of allogeneic haematopoietic stem cells [8,9,15]. The feasibility has been greatly improved since the introduction of reduced or non-myeloablative conditioning regimens [9]. The success of allogeneic stem cell transplantation is also dependent on the level of cytoreduction achieved by the induction chemotherapy as immunological effects leading to the graft-versus-myeloma (GvM) effect need several months to take place. Cytoreduction before allogeneic SCT is particularly relevant for reduced conditioning regimens as in many patients the achievement of complete donor chimerism is a gradual process that can take several months [9,15].

An anti-myeloma effect of thalidomide alone has been demonstrated in several clinical trails [12,19,21]. Recent data indicate that thalidomide, which has antiangiogenic properties, can increase the therapeutic effect of chemotherapy and might contribute to overcome drug resistance [5,11,17,18]. Therefore we investigated therapeutic efficacy and feasibility of a treatment regimen combining thalidomide, cyclophosphamide, etoposide and dexamethasone (TCED) in poor-prognosis multiple myeloma.

Materials and methods

Fifty-six patients with poor-prognosis MM were included in a phase II clinical protocol (TCED protocol): primary refractory to conventional chemotherapy (n = 5), secondary refractory to conventional chemotherapy (n = 17), resistant relapse and untested relapse after autologous blood stem cell transplantation (n = 16), plasma cell leukaemia (n = 1). The study protocol was approved by the institutional review boards. Thalidomide treatment (400 mg taken at night time p.o.) was continued until toxic side effects, progression or another event occurred that led to the exclusion of the patient from the study. CED chemotherapy (cyclophosphamide 400 mg/m^2 i.v. and etoposide 40 mg/m^2 both i.v. as continuous infusion day 1–4; dexamethasone 40 mg p.o. day 1–4; repeat after 28 days) was given for 3 to a maximum of 6 cycles until best response. Patients received daily prophylactic antibiotic treatment. To reduce the number of leukopenic days after chemotherapy, subcutaneous administration of G-CSF (Neupogen, Amgen Coop., USA) was recommended, starting on day seven after the start of chemotherapy in a dose of 300 μg for patients up to 75 kg body weight, or 480 μg above 75 kg body weight.

Primary end point of the study was the response to TCED therapy. Response criteria were used according to guidelines of the EBMT/IBMTR [3].

All patients, irrespective of the duration of therapy, were included in the evaluation of adverse effects. The system of classification of the World Health Organization was used.

Events excluding from progression-free survival (PFS) were death from any cause and progressive disease. Estimates of PFS and overall survival (OAS) distributions were calculated according to the method of Kaplan and Meier [13]. Statistical computations were performed using the software packages S-Plus (MathSoft, Inc., Seattle, USA), and StatXact4 for Windows (Cytel Software Corp., Cambridge, USA).

Results

Our study focused on the treatment of a collective of pretreated MM patients with adverse prognostic factors. 87.5% of patients had a stage III according to Durie and Salmon, and beta2-microglobulin levels were above the upper limit of normal range of 2.4 mg/dl in 76.7% of patients. Six patients were not evaluable for response, as therapy could not be continued after the first cycle of chemotherapy for the following reasons: intolerance to thalidomide (4 patients), sudden cardiac death (1 patient at day 36 after start of thalidomide with a previous history of ischemic heart disease and tachyarrhythmia absoluta), septic death (1 patient). In the 50 remaining patients a median number of 3 cycles (range 3 to 6 cycles) were given to achieve maximal response to treatment. We recorded 4% (n = 2) complete responses (CR), 64% (n = 32) partial responses (PR), 18% (n = 9) minimal responses (MR), 6% (n = 3) stable diseases (SD), 8% (4) progressive diseases (PD) resulting in a response rate (>/= MR) of 86.6% (for n = 50 patients evaluable for response). According to an intend-to-treat analysis the overall objective response rate (n = 56) was 76.7%.

The response to TCED treatment was consolidated in 18 patients by ABSCT (n = 9) or allogeneic stem cell transplantation (n = 9). The observation time of these 18 patients was censored at the time of transplantation for calculation of progression-free-survival. In one patient we were able to harvest an autologous stem cell transplant in the G-CSF supported period of haematopoietic recovery after the second cycle of TCED.

Survival time estimation was done on an intention-to-treat basis for all 56 patients. The estimated median follow-up duration was 14 months. The median PFS was 16 months (Fig. 4.2-1). The estimated 1-year progression-free survival was 60.2% (95% CI 0.41 to 0.75). The median OAS time has not been reached so far. The last observed death was after 16 months of follow-up. The estimated survival probability is 55%. The estimated 1-year overall survival for all 56 patients was 62.6% (95% CI 46.8% to 75%). Using the log-rank test to analyse the relationship of response and overall survival, the estimated hazard ratio of non-responders (n = 7) compared to responders (n = 43) was 4.1 showing a significant survival benefit for responding patients (95% CI 1.5 to 11.6; p = 0.005).

Using the Cox proportional hazards model in a univariant analysis overall survival was positively correlated with less than 50% plasma cell infiltration in the bone marrow (p = 0.04; n = 41) and duration of intake of full-dose thalidomide (p = 0.08; n = 56). Other parameters (beta2-microglobulin, age and

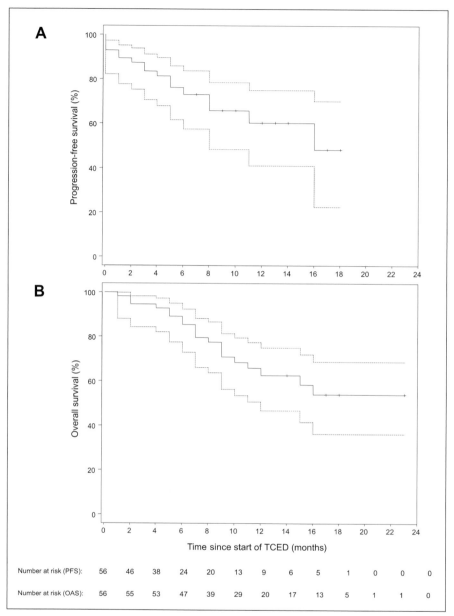

Figure 4.2-1A,B Kaplan-Meier curves of (A) PFS (median of 16 months) and (B) OAS (median 12+ months) for all 56 patients included in the study.

previous therapy) did not show a significant correlation to PFS, OAS or response to therapy.

Thalidomide-associated WHO grade I and II adverse effects were in the same range as reported previously, including somnolence (32%), constipation (28%), tingling or numbness (23%), weakness (12%), tremors (11%), dizziness (10%) [8,9,22]. Adverse effects attributed to thalidomide resulted in a dose reduction

Table 4.2-1 Incidence of WHO-grade III and IV toxicities (n = 56).

Adverse effects	No. of patients (%)
Leukocytopenia (< 1.0/nl)	32 (74.0)[1]
Thrombocytopenia (< 20/nl)	9 (20.9)[1]
Severe infection	20 (35.7)[2]
Transfusion requirement	
RBC[4]	28 (50.0)
Thrombocytes	8 (14.2)
Cardiovascular	4 (7.1)[3]
Tingling or numbness	3 (5.3)
Hearing disturbance	1 (1.7)
Acute psychosis	1 (1.7)
Constipation (subileus)	1 (1.7)

[1] Total of 43 patients evaluable
[2] Infection requiring hospitalization and i.v. antibiotic treatment and one of the following criteria: organ infection (e.g. pneumonia), positive blood cultures, infection of central venous catheter, death due to infectious complications
[3] Sudden death (cardiac arrest), AV-Block grade II requiring cardiac pacemaker, thrombosis of v. subclavia, deep vein thrombosis
[4] RBC = red blood cells

in 55% and discontinuation of thalidomide in 19.6% of patients. Major WHO III and IV toxicities were infections (35%) and cardiovascular events (7.1%) (see Table 4.2-1).

Discussion

The rationale to use the CED regimen in combination with thalidomide in our study was to avoid potential cross resistance to anthracyclines or melphalan, often used in first-line therapy of MM, and usage of chemotherapeutic agents with established activity in relapse MM patients [1,2,6,14,20]. The CED regimen has a lower incidence of neurological and renal toxicity compared with other second line regimens [4,7,16,22]. This is of importance, as we intended to avoid cumulative neurological toxicity in combination with thalidomide. The lower dosage of chemotherapeutics in comparison to previous studies using CED regimens was chosen, and application of additional chemotherapeutic agents was avoided since our protocol included elderly and heavily pretreated patients with increased susceptibility to haematological and infectious complications. Consequently, dexamethasone was applied only in the first 4 days of each cycle and not between individual cycles as in other protocols [2]. This was justified as the major benefit of our protocol was considered to result from the combination of CED with thalidomide.

Because of patient heterogeneity, it is difficult to directly compare the results of our trial with previous studies using conventional and high-dose therapy for poor-prognosis MM. In eligible patients with relapsed or refractory MM best treatment results are achieved with ABSCT [14] inducing overall response rates of 58% (CR and PR) with a median progression-free survival of 11 months and an overall survival of 19 months [22].

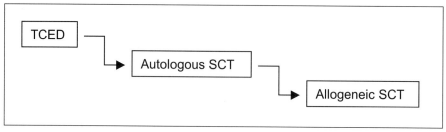

Figure 4.2-2 Schematic representation of an aggressive treatment strategy to induce long-term remissions in eligible patients with poor-prognosis multiple myeloma

Our study indicates an at least equivalent therapeutic efficacy of TCED as reported for conventional chemotherapy and ABSCT for this group of patients. Our results encourage future studies to evaluate the role of thalidomide in combination with chemotherapeutic regimens in MM and other oncological entities.

The described therapeutic efficiency, as well as the possibility for stem cell harvest in the haematopoietic recovery phase after each cycle, qualify the TCED regimen as a very good regimen for remission induction in patients with poor-prognosis MM eligible for autologous or allogeneic SCT.

Consequently, for eligible patients below the age of 65 years, we propose a study design that operates with the sequential application of three cycles of TCED followed by autologous SCT and consolidation by non-myeloablative allogeneic SCT (Fig. 4.2-2).

Acknowledgements

We wish to thank Dr. Sehlbach, Duisburg, and Dr. U. Hegenbart, Leipzig, for support in data accrual. We thank Dr. K. Zwingenberger, Gruenenhal GmbH, Aachen, Germany, for providing thalidomide.

References

1. ALEXANIAN, R., M. DIMOPOULOS: The treament of Multiple Myeloma. N Engl J Med 330 (1994) 484–489.
2. BARLOGIE, B., et al.: Effective treatment of advanced multiple myeloma refractory to alkylating agents. N Engl J Med 310 (1984) 1353–1356.
3. BLADE, J., et al.: Criteria for definition of response, relapse and progression in multiple myeloma after high-dose therapy. Br J Haematol 102 (1998) 1115–1123.
4. BONNET, J.D., et al.: Addition of cisplatin and bleomycin to vincristin-carmustine-doxorubicin-prednison (VBAP) combination in the treatment of relapsing or resistant multiple myeloma: a Southwest Oncology Group study. Cancer Treat Rep 68 (1984) 481–485.
5. D'AMATO, R.J., et al.: Thalidomide is an inhibitor of angiogenesis. Proc Natl Acad Sci USA 91 (1994) 4082–4085.
6. DIMOPOULOS, M.A., et al.: Cyclophosphamide and etoposide therapy with GM-CSF for VAD resistant multiple myeloma. Br J Haematol 83 (1993) 240–244.
7. DIMOPOULOS, M.A., et al.: Primary therapy of multiple myeloma with paclitaxel (taxol). Ann Oncol 5 (1994) 757–759.

8. GHARTON, G., *et al.*: Allogeneic bone marrow transplantation in multiple myeloma: an update of the EBMT registry. VIth International Workshop on Multiple Myeloma. Syllabus, Boston, MA, (1997) June 14–18.

9. GIRALT, S,. *et al.*: Non-myeloablative conditioning with fludarabine (F)/melphalan (M) for patients with multiple myeloma (MM). Am Soc Clin Oncol 18 (1999) 6a.

10. GOLDSCHMIDT, H., *et al.*: High-dose therapy with peripheral blood progenitor cell transplantation in multiple myeloma. Annal Oncol 8 (1997) 243–246.

11. HIDESHIMA, T., *et al.*: Thalidomide and its analogs overcome drug resistance of human multiple myeloma cells to conventional therapy. Blood 96 (2000) 2943–2950.

12. JULIUSSON, G., *et al.*: Frequent good partial remission from Thalidomide including best response ever in patients with advanced refractory and relapsed multiple myeloma. Br J Haematol 108 (2000) 229–2230.

13. KAPLAN, E.L., and P. MEIER: Nonparametric estimation from incomplete observations. J Am Stat Assoc 53 (1958) 457–481.

14. KYLE, R.A.: Diagnosis and management of multiple myeloma and related disorders. Prog Haematol 14 (1996) 257–282.

15. LOKHORST, H.M., *et al.*: Donor leukocyte infusions are effective in relapsed multiple myeloma after allogeneic bone marrow transplantation. Blood 90 (1997) 4206–4211.

16. MILLER, H. *et al.*: Paclitaxel as the initial treatment of multiple myeloma: an Eastern Cooperative Oncology Group Study. Am J Clin Oncol 21 (1998) 553–556.

17. MOEHLER, T.M., *et al.*: Thalidomide and CED chemotherapy as salvage therapy in poor prognosis multiple myeloma. Blood 101 (2000) 290b.

18. MUNSHI, N., *et al.*: Chemotherapy with DT-PACE for previously treated multiple myeloma. Blood 94 (1999) Suppl. 1 123a,.

19. NEBEN, K., *et al.*: High plasma basic fibroblast growth factor (bFGF) concentration is associated with good response to Thalidomide monotherapy in progressive multiple myeloma. Blood 101 (2000) 124a.

20. SAN MIGUEL, J.F., *et al.*: Treatment of multiple myeloma. Haematologica 84 (1999) 36–58.

21. SINGHAL, S., *et al.*: Antitumor activity of Thalidomide in refractory multiple myeloma. N Engl J Med 341 (1999) 1565–1571.

22. VESOLE, D.H., *et al.*: High-dose Melphalan with autotransplantation for refractory multiple myeloma: results of a southwest oncology group phase II trial. J Clin Oncol 17 (1999) 2173–2179.

4.3 Anti-CD20 Monoclonal Antibody (Rituximab) in Combination with Cytotoxic Chemotherapy for the Treatment of Follicular Lymphoma

Martin, S., R. Kronenwett, A. Niederste-Hollenberg, I. Mlynarczuk, G. Meckenstock, R. Haas

Dept. of Hematology, Oncology and Clinical Immunology
University of Düsseldorf, Germany

Summary

Eradication of minimal residual disease in patients with follicular non-Hodgkin's lymphoma is rarely seen after chemotherapy alone. The anti-CD20 monoclonal antibody Rituximab represents a new therapeutic tool for patients with B-cell lymphoma, since it targets an antigen restricted to the B-cell lineage, expressed by over 95% of the lymphoma cells. Our study shows the efficacy of Rituximab combined with cytotoxic chemotherapy in inducing clinical and molecular remissions in patients with follicular lymphoma. The rationale for this therapeutic strategy relies on the efficacy of Rituximab as single agent in lymphoma patients, non-cross resistant mechanisms of action and *in vitro* synergy with cytotoxic agents.

Introduction

Historically, patients with follicular lymphoma are not cured by conventional chemotherapy. Despite an initial high response rate, the clinical course consists of a pattern of repeated relapses, and most patients ultimately develop refractory disease or transformation into an aggressive lymphoma. Treatment with myeloablative therapy and stem cell support significantly improved the prognosis of patients with advanced-stage follicular lymphoma, especially when transplanted early in the course of the disease [11,12]. In our experience with high-dose therapy and autologous peripheral blood stem cell transplantation in 111 patients, the probability of relapse-free survival at 4 years after transplantation was 78% for patients treated in first remission [23].

In the arsenal of lymphoma therapy, the anti-CD20 monoclonal antibody Rituximab provides a new treatment option, with an anti-tumour effect different from the cell-kill mechanisms exerted by cytotoxic drugs. Rituximab is the first MoAb approved by the Federal Drug Administration (FDA) for the treatment of follicular lymphoma. It is a genetically engineered chimeric anti-CD20 monoclonal antibody (MoAb) containing human IgG_1 and κ constant regions with murine variable regions [19]. The CD20 molecule, a tetraspan membrane-associated phosphoprotein which serves as calcium channel, initiates intracellular signals and modulates G_1/S cell cycle progression [21,22], provides an ideal target for treatment of lymphomas with MoAb. This relies on its expression restricted to the B-cell lineage and presence on over 95% of non-Hodgkin's lymphoma cells [26]. The antigen is not down-regulated, internalized

Figure 4.3-1A,B The t(14;18) translocation.
A: Schematic representation of the reciprocal translocation between chromosomes 14 and 18.
B: Schematic representation of the VDJ region of the Ig heavy-chain gene on chromosome 14, of the *bcl-2* gene on chromosome 18 and of the *bcl-2/IgH* fusion as a consequence of the translocation.

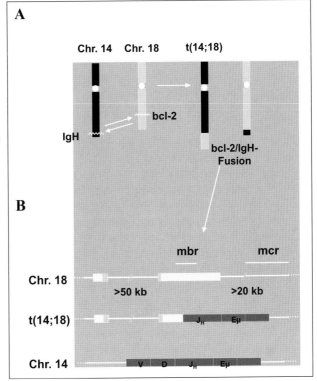

or shed in response to stimulation [19,21]. The mechanism of action of Rituximab is based on complement-dependent cytotoxicity [8] and antibody-dependent cell-mediated cytotoxicity [2]. In addition, extensive crosslinking of CD20 leads to direct cell death by induction of apoptosis [20]. In clinical trials, using Rituximab as single agent, while well tolerated, the antibody induced a rapid depletion of CD20-positive normal B-cells and lymphoma cells, with response rates between 32% and 62% in patients with relapsed follicular lymphoma, mantle cell and diffuse large-cell lymphoma [3,6,15,16,17]. The high response rate in chemotherapy-refractory patients and the favourable toxicity profile prompted the administration of Rituximab as first-line therapy in patients with low-grade non-Hodgkin's lymphoma. HAINSWORTH et al. [13] observed a response rate of 64%, including 23% complete remissions, in a group of 41 patients. Since drug-resistant lymphoma cells become sensitive to cytotoxic agents after *in vitro* treatment with Rituximab [5], an additional therapeutic benefit was envisaged by combining the anti-CD20 antibody with cytotoxic chemotherapy. Indeed, the favourable effect of chemo-immunotherapy was mirrored by a response rate of 95%, with 55% complete remissions [4].

Follicular lymphoma is characterized in about 80% of cases by the chromosomal translocation t(14;18), juxtaposing the *bcl-2* oncogene on chromosome 18 with a J_H segment of the immunoglobulin heavy-chain gene on chromosome 14 [1] (Fig. 4.3-1). As a consequence of the translocation, *bcl-2* is overexpressed, and the antiapoptotic BCL-2 protein accumulates in the cell. While localized in the outer mitochondrial membrane, endoplasmic reticulum and the nuclear membrane [14], BCL-2 in interaction with the death agonists confers the affected cell a survival advantage [25].

Using a nested polymerase chain reaction (PCR), cells harbouring the *bcl-2* gene rearrangement can be identified, which allows detection of "minimal residual disease" [9].

The aim of our currently performed study is to assess the efficacy of Rituximab when given in combination with cytotoxic chemotherapy in patients with follicular lymphoma. Taking advantage of the molecular tools to assess minimal residual disease, we were interested in evaluating the ability of Rituximab plus high-dose cytosine-arabinoside and mitoxantrone (HAM) to induce molecular remissions in patients with follicular lymphoma.

Patients and methods

Patients

Patients were eligible for the study if they had a CD20-positive follicular lymphoma according to the REAL classification and carried the t(14;18) translocation in peripheral blood and/or bone marrow. Thirteen patients with failure of previous therapy, or newly diagnosed patients with advanced-stage disease, were included. The requirement of therapy was defined as progressive disease of $> 50\%$ during the last six months, presence of B-symptoms, bone marrow infiltration resulting in cytopenia or bulky disease.

Treatment

Independent of the disease status, the patients received high-dose cytarabine (2 g/m^2 q 12 h on days 1 and 2) and mitoxantrone (10 mg/m^2/day on days 2 and 3). For up-front patients, this regimen was given as consolidation after first-line cytotoxic therapy, while patients enrolled at relapse after conventional therapy were treated with HAM as salvage regimen. In addition to its anti-tumour effect, this regimen also served in both groups for stem cell mobilization. Rituximab (375 mg/m^2) was administered as intravenous infusion one day before the HAM cycle. Oral premedication with an antipyretic and an antihistamine was given, but no steroids were administered. Patients considered to be at risk of tumour-lysis syndrome received prophylactic allopurinol and hydration. If toxicity occurred in the form of hypotension, rigors, mucosal congestion or oedema, bronchospasm or any other medically significant event, the infusion was temporarily discontinued. Infusions were restarted at 50% of the previous rate and then escalated as tolerated.

Granulocyte colony-stimulating factor (G-CSF, Neupogen, Amgen, Thousand Oaks, CA, USA) was commenced 24 h after the completion of cytotoxic chemotherapy at a daily dose of 300 μg, s.c. Peripheral blood stem cell (PBSC) harvesting began when a distinct population of CD34$^+$ cells was detectable by immunofluorescence analysis in peripheral blood. Leukaphereses were performed using a Spectra device (Cobe Laboratories, Lakewood, CA, USA) by processing 20 l of blood at flow rates of 70–150 ml/min.

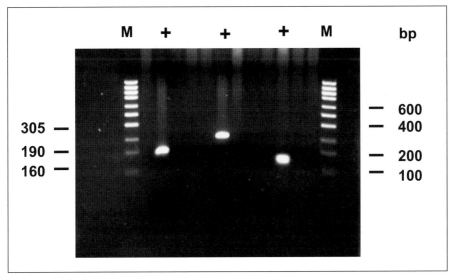

Figure 4.3-2 Analysis by gel-electrophoresis of 12 samples after nested PCR. The size of the positive (+) probes is indicated. M = 100-bp marker.

Molecular analysis of bcl–2/IgH rearrangement

Mononuclear cells from peripheral blood (PB), bone marrow (BM) and leukapheresis (LP) products were obtained following separation by Ficoll (Biochrom, Berlin, Germany). Genomic DNA was extracted using the QIAmp DNA Blood Mini Kit (QIAGEN GmbH, Hilden, Germany) following the manufacturer's instructions.

Molecular monitoring was accomplished using a nested-primer assay performed at the major breakpoint region (MBR) or minor cluster region (mcr) of the *bcl–2/IgH* locus. One μg of genomic DNA was amplified using the primers described by GRIBBEN *et al.* [9].

The sensitivity of the nested PCR obtained by diluting the t(14;18)-positive cell line K422 (DSMZ, Deutsche Sammlung für Mikroorganismen und Zellkulturen, Braunschweig, Germany) in t(14;18)-negative normal mono-nuclear cells was one t(14;18)-positive cell in 10^5–10^6 control cells.

Aliquots of the final reaction were analysed by electrophoresis in 2% agarose gel containing ethidium bromide in tris-borate electrophoresis buffer and visualized under UV light (Fig. 4.3-2).

Results and discussion

In our study, all patients treated with Rituximab/HAM had objective responses, yielding therefore an overall response rate of 100%. In 69% of the patients a complete remission was documented, whereas the proportion of patients achieving only a partial remission after the combined chemo-immunotherapy was 31%. As far as the latter group is concerned, nodal residual disease persisted in all but one patient with regressive splenomegaly. On the other hand, none of the patients had residual marrow infiltration as documented by histological examination, inferring a better drug accessibility of bone marrow. Conceivably, the tumour cell depletion may reflect a gradient of antibody distribution that decreases from peripheral blood through bone marrow to lymph nodes.

The favourable experience with Rituximab in pre-treated patients as reported by several groups [3,6,15,16,17], suggested that the antibody efficacy is not affected by prior exposure to cytotoxic chemotherapy. In this respect, our results would support a more nuanced relationship between response and disease history. Despite the high overall response rate that we also observed, a more detailed analysis of the quality of the remission achieved showed a better response in chemotherapy-naive patients, since 80% of them had a complete remission following Rituximab/HAM. Differently, failure to respond to prior therapies was associated with a "poorer" response to Rituximab/HAM, as only half of the patients treated at relapse had no evidence of disease according to clinical and histopathological restaging examinations, whereas the other half achieved "only" partial remission.

Even when inducing transient clinical complete remissions, standard-dose cytotoxic regimens such as CHOP (cyclophosphamide, doxorubicin, vincristine, prednison) are not able to eradicate minimal residual disease. This is documented by the persistence of cells bearing the bcl-2/IgH rearrangement in bone marrow or peripheral blood following therapy [10]. Residual chemoresistant lymphoma cells may be responsible for relapse. The presence of PCR-detectable cells in the bone marrow or peripheral blood of patients in clinical remission, after conventional chemotherapy or after high-dose therapy, may be predictive for disease recurrence. In a group of 47 patients with follicular lymphoma who underwent a myeloablative therapy with peripheral blood stem cell support, we found a positive PCR-result at any point of time after transplantation. This would indicate a 4.5-fold greater relative risk of developing a relapse when compared to a negative PCR result [18]. In the same line of thoughts, FREEDMAN et al. [7] demonstrated a strong relationship between the probability of disease-free survival and the PCR status obtained from bone marrow samples after transplantation. In particular, they found that continued PCR-negativity in follow-up samples is highly predictive for continuous complete remission. In addition, patients whose autografts were free of tumour cells experienced a significantly longer freedom from recurrence than those transplanted with t(14;18)-positive leukapheresis products, as reflected in a probability of relapse-free survival of 82% versus 20% after a follow-up time of 12 years.

All patients included in our study had a t(14;18)-positive follicular lymphoma, as proved by molecular diagnostic before the start of treatment. Using PCR to assess the frequency of involvement with lymphoma, we observed a dissemination pattern between the two haematopoietic compartments, i.e. bone marrow and peripheral blood, dependent on the disease history. In newly diagnosed patients, peripheral blood was the compartment more often affected, whereas bone marrow was always positive for bcl-2/IgH rearrangement-bearing cells in patients with a relapse following previous therapy.

Follow-up samples were available for all patients allowing the evaluation of "molecular response", which we defined as the conversion from PCR-positivity to a PCR-negative status after therapy.

As shown by molecular monitoring, the combination of Rituximab and HAM is capable of clearing lymphoma from blood and marrow. When the molecular response was evaluated in the context of clinical response, a significant correlation was found between the molecular status and the result of clinical staging after therapy, i.e. none of the patients who remained PCR-positive had a clinical complete remission.

The therapeutic benefit of the combined Rituximab/HAM treatment, with respect to residual tumour cells in leukapheresis products, is convincingly reflected by the comparison with the results obtained with HAM chemotherapy alone. In our experience, in 47 patients treated with the same regimen without Rituximab, PCR-positivity persisted in 74% of the leukapheresis products. In the current study, we confirmed our previous results [24] in 7 patients with follicular lymphoma, since, after addition of the MoAb, only 15% of the autografts collected still remained contaminated with tumour cells. As a result, and comparing the efficacy of the two regimens, i.e. HAM with or without Rituximab, to yield lymphoma-free harvests, the Rituximab/HAM combination is clearly superior. The substantial anti-tumour effect without causing additional toxicity is an exciting clinical success. Rituximab plus high-dose cytarabine/mitoxantrone yields harvests which, in patients receiving this therapy as first-line or salvage treatment, are free of tumour cells. Supported by G-CSF, Rituximab/HAM is also an effective regimen to mobilize PBSC.

The depletion of B-cells from peripheral blood and bone marrow with Rituximab/HAM, with an attendant negative PCR result, represents an advantageous *in vivo* purging, which minimizes the tumour cell contamination of stem cell harvests and obviates the need for *ex vivo* selection procedures. Since patients given this dose-escalated regimen are envisaged for a high-dose therapy with autologous peripheral blood stem cell support, the *in vivo* purging, prior to impending stem cell transplantation, also provides the advantage of "priming" the residual lymphoma cells by antibody exposure, in order to become more chemosensitive to the conditioning regimen.

In conclusion, the eradication of t(14;18)-positive cells in patients with clinical complete remission suggests that Rituximab/HAM significantly reduces tumour burden, even under the threshold of minimal residual disease detection. This is true for newly diagnosed patients as well as for patients eligible for second-line therapy. Given our previous results [18], notably, the achievement of a durable molecular remission may lead to prolonged disease-free survival.

References

1. BAKHSHI, A., et al.: Cloning the chromosomal breakpoint of t(14;18) human lymphomas: clustering around JH on chromosome 14 and near a transcriptional unit on 18. Cell 41 (1985) 899.
2. CLYNES, R.A., et al.: Inhibitory Fc receptors modulate in vivo cytotoxicity against tumour targets. Nature Medicine 6 (2000) 443.
3. COIFFIER, B., et al.: Rituximab (anti-CD20 monoclonal antibody) for the treatment of patients with relapsing or refractory aggressive lymphoma: A multicenter phase II study. Blood 92 (1998) 1927.

4. CZUCZMAN, M.S., *et al.*: Treatment of patients with low-grade B-cell lymphoma with the combination of chimeric anti-CD20 monoclonal antibody and CHOP chemotherapy. J Clin Oncol 17 (1999) 268.

5. DEMIDEM, A., *et al.*: Chimeric anti-CD20 (IDEC-C2B8) monoclonal antibody sensitizes a B-cell lymphoma cell line to cell killing by cytotoxic drugs. Cancer Biother and Radiopharm 12 (1997) 177.

6. FORAN, J.M., *et al.*: European phase II study of Rituximab (chimeric anti-CD20 monoclonal antibody) for patients with newly diagnosed mantle-cell lymphoma and previously treated mantle-cell lymphoma, immunocytoma and small B-cell lymphocytic lymphoma. J Clin Oncol 18 (2000) 317.

7. FREEDMAN, A.S., *et al.*: Long-term follow-up of autologous bone marrow transplantation in patients with relapsed follicular lymphoma. Blood 94 (1999) 3325.

8. GOLAY, J., *et al.*: Biologic response of B-lymphoma cells to anti-CD20 monoclonal antibody rituximab in vitro: CD55 and CD59 regulate complement-mediated cell lysis. Blood 95 (2000) 3900.

9. GRIBBEN, J.G., *et al.*: Detection by polymerase chain reaction of residual cells with the bcl-2 translocation is associated with increased risk of relapse after autologous bone marrow transplantation for B-cell lymphoma. Blood 81 (1993) 3449.

10. GRIBBEN, J., *et al.*: All advanced-stage non-Hodgkin's lymphomas with a polymerase chain reaction amplifiable breakpoint of BCL-2 have residual cells containing the BCL-2 rearrangement at evaluation and after treatment. Blood 78 (1991) 3275.

11. HAAS, R., *et al.*: Patient characteristics associated with successful mobilizing and autografting of peripheral blood progenitor cells in malignant lymphoma. Blood 83 (1994) 3787.

12. HAAS, R., *et al.*: Sequential high-dose therapy with peripheral blood progenitor cell support in low-grade Non-Hodgkin lymphoma. J Clin Oncol 12 (1994) 1685.

13. HAINSWORTH, J.D., *et al.*: Rituximab monoclonal antibody as initial systemic therapy for patients with low-grade non-Hodgkin lymphoma. Blood 95 (2000), 3052.

14. KRAJEWSKI, S., *et al.*: Investigation of the subcellular distribution of the BCL-2 oncoprotein: Residence in the nuclear envelope, endoplasmic reticulum, and outer mitochondrial membranes. Cancer Res 53 (1993) 4701.

15. MALONEY, D.G., *et al.*: Phase I clinical trial using escalating single-dose infusion of chimeric anti-CD20 monoclonal antibody (IDEC-C2B8) in patients with recurrent B-cell lymphoma. Blood 84 (1994) 2457.

16. MALONEY, D.G., *et al.*: IDEC-C2B8 (Rituximab) anti-CD20 monoclonal antibody therapy in patients with relapsed low-grade non-Hodgkin's lymphoma. Blood 90 (1997) 2188.

17. MCLAUGHLIN, P., *et al.*: Rituximab chimeric anti-CD20 monoclonal antibody therapy for relapsed indolent lymphoma: half of patients respond to a four-dose treatment program. J Clin Oncol 16 (1998) 2825.

18. MOOS, M., *et al.*: The remission status before and the PCR status after high-dose therapy with peripheral blood stem cell support are prognostic factors for relapse-free survival in patients with follicular non-Hodgkin's lymphoma. Leukemia 12 (1998) 1971.

19. REFF, M.E., *et al.*: Depletion of B-cells in vivo by a chimeric mouse human monoclonal antibody to CD20. Blood 83 (1994) 435.

20. SHAN, D., *et al.*: Apoptosis of malignant human B cells by ligation of CD20 with monoclonal antibodies. Blood 91 (1998) 1644.

21. TEDDER, T.F., ENGEL, P.: CD20: a regulator of cell cycle progression of B-lymphocytes. Immunol Today 15 (1994) 450.

22. TEDDER, T.F., *et al.*: Antibodies reactive with the B1 molecule inhibit cell cycle progression but not activation of human B lymphocytes. Eur J Immunol 16 (1986) 881.

23. VOSO, M.T., *et al.*: Prognostic factors for the clinical outcome of patients with follicular lymphoma following high-dose therapy and peripheral blood stem cell transplantation (PBSCT). Bone Marrow Transplant. 25 (2000) 957.

24. VOSO, M.T., *et al.*: In vivo depletion of B cells using a combination of high-dose cytosine-arabinoside/mitoxantrone and rituximab for autografting in patients with non-Hodgkin's lymphoma. BJH 109, 729–735, 2000.

25. YANG, E., KORSMEYER, S.J.: Molecular thanatopsis: A discourse on the BCL2 family and cell death. Blood 88 (1996) 386.

26. ZHOU, L.J., *et al.*: CD20 Workshop Panel Report. In: Schlossmann, S.F., Bournsell, L., Gilks, W., *et al.* (Eds.): Leukocyte typing V. White cell differentiation antigens. Oxford University, Oxford UK (1995) 511–514.

4.4 Mobilization of Peripheral Blood Progenitor Cells (PBPC) in Normal Donors for Allogeneic PBPC Transplantation: Comparison between Once a Day versus Twice a Day G-CSF Administration - A Retrospective Analysis

Pönisch, W., S. Leiblein*, E. Edel, B. Haustein, J. Leupold,
U. Hegenbart, C. Becker, T. Lange, F. Riese, J. Möckel, H. K. Al-Ali,
C. Kliem, L. Uharek, D. Niederwieser

Dept. of Haematology/Oncology, University of Leipzig, Leipzig, Germany

* To whom correspondence should be addressed (leibs@medizin.uni-leipzig.de)

Summary

Between January 1995 and March 2000, we collected peripheral blood progenitor cells from 124 healthy donors (age: 17–72 years), mobilized with rhG-CSF (group 1 included 91 donors receiving 2 x 5 μg/kg/day s.c. for 3 days and group 2 included 33 donors receiving 1 x 15 μg/kg/day s.c. for 5 days). In a retrospective analysis we compared two different schedules of G-CSF application. Our results suggest that administration of G-CSF in normal donors at doses of 2 x 5 μg/kg/day mobilizes significantly more progenitor cells than 1 x 15 μg/kg/day given in a single dose, thus making an earlier apheresis (at day 3 or 4) possible and reducing the required sessions. In general, the observed side effects were acceptable.

Introduction

The use of allogeneic peripheral blood progenitor cells (PBPC) in haemato-poietic stem cell transplantations has significantly increased over the last few years [4]. Allogeneic peripheral blood progenitor cell transplantation (PBPCT) may have benefits for both donor and recipient. The advantages of PBPC collection are the absence of general anaesthesia for the donor, the possibility of collecting more stem cells, and the possibility of harvesting the cells in an outpatient setting. The recipients may experience a more rapid recovery of haematopoiesis and of the immune system, which would reduce treatment-related morbidity, facilitate earlier discharge from hospital, and decrease costs.

Peripheral stem cells can be isolated with few separations in healthy donors, out of the steady state, after a short course of stimulation with haematopoietic growth factors like recombinant human granulocyte-colony stimulating factor (rhG-CSF). Different protocols with respect to dose and duration of the G-CSF application are currently in use. The optimal G-CSF dose and schedule would ensure the collection of an adequate PBPC number while minimizing donors' cytokine exposure and side effects. This dose has not been established, partly because the optimal PBPC dose required for engraftment and overall transplant outcome is unknown. The majority of published data used a dose of 5–10 μg/kg body weight G-CSF in a single subcutaneous administration over 5–7 consecutive days and 2 separations [2,3,7,10].

An administration schedule of twice a day has been used by some groups [1,2]. The rationale for a twice daily schedule is based on the fact that the elimination half-life of rhG-CSF, after subcutaneous or intravenous administration, is only about 3 to 4 hours [6,8]. However, the biological half-life of rhG-CSF is known to be significantly longer [6,9]. Mobilization and transplantation results appear similar with either daily or twice daily rhG-CSF administration schedules.

In this retrospective analysis, we have compared two different schedules of rhG-CSF for mobilization of PBPC in normal donors, including a single daily dose of 15 μg/kg/day for 5 days *versus* a dose of 5 μg/kg/twice daily for 3 days. We have determined the number of leukocytes and CD34+ cells in mobilized peripheral blood, the number of aphereses needed to obtain the target dose, the apheresis products as well as the side effects.

Materials and methods

Normal donors

Between January 1995 and March 2000 we collected peripheral blood progenitor cells from 124 healthy HLA-matched donors mobilized with rhG-CSF (Neupogen®) (Table 4.4-1). Protocols for collection of PBPC were approved by the local Ethics Committee, and written informed consent was obtained from every donor before the procedure. PBPC collections were used for either HLA identical related (n = 112) or unrelated (n = 12) allogeneic transplants.

Mobilization and apheresis

Normal donors received G-CSF according to two different schedules in a consecutive way: group 1 included 91 donors treated with 2 x 5 μg/kg/day s.c. for 3 days and group 2 in which 33 donors were treated with 1 x 15 μg/kg/day s.c. for 5 days. Adverse events were graded by WHO toxicity criteria.

We collected PBPC from 3–5 fold blood volume. Leukaphereses were performed with a CS 3000 Plus (Baxter) or a COBE Spectra (COBE) cell separator using cubital veins. Each session lasted approximately 4 hours. Leukapheresis products were analysed as follows: total and differential cell count, CD34+ cell estimation and CFU-GM assay. At least 4 x 10^6 CD34+ cells/kg body weight of the recipient had to be collected.

Apheresis products were infused within 24 hours.

Table 4.4-1 Donor characteristics and days of aphereses.

		Group 1 (2 x 5 μg/kg/day)	Group 2 (1 x 15 μg/kg/day)	p value
Number of donors		91	33	
Age (median) range		41(17–60)	46(19–72)	n.s.
Gender (m/f)		58/33	13/20	P < 0.03
Number of aphereses:	1	41	14	
	2	50	17	n.s.
	3	0	2	

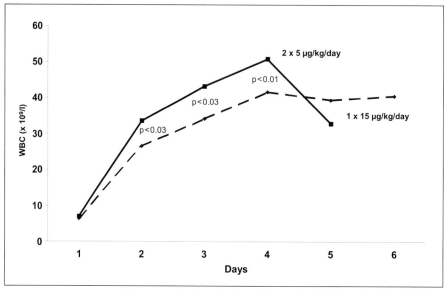

Figure 4.4-1 Increase of WBC in healthy donors after 2 x 5 µg/kg/day rhG-CSF on days 1–3 or 1 x 15 µg/kg/day rhG-CSF on days 1–5.

Mononuclear cell determination

Mononuclear cell determination was performed in apheresis products. The total cell count was determined by a Coulter counter. A manual 200 cell differential count was also obtained. Mononuclear cells included lymphocytes, blasts, monocytes, promyelocytes, myelocytes and metamyelocytes.

Analysis of CD34 positive cells

Samples (blood and apheresis products) were phenotyped by a lysed whole blood technique [5]. 100 µl (cells diluted to approximately 10^7/ml) were incubated with a mixture of 20 µl anti-CD45-FITC (clone 2D1) and 20 µl CD34-PE (clone 8G12) or isotype control (Becton Dickinson) for 15 min at room temperature. Erythrocytes were lysed by addition of 2 ml FACS Lysing Solution (Becton Dickinson) for 10 min. The samples were washed with PBS/azide, resuspended in PBS with 1 % formaldehyde and analysed immediately by flow cytometry (FACScan, Becton Dickinson). Fifty thousand events were collected as list mode data. Analysis was done according to the directions of the working group "Flow Cytometry" of DGTI.

Analysis of CFU-GM

Cultures were set up in methylcellulose medium (Methocult H4443, Stem Cell Technologies Inc.) supplemented with 50 IU rhG-CSF/ml. Cells were cultured at 10^5/ml in 35 x 10 mm Petri dishes. The colonies (more than 50 cells) were scored on day 10.

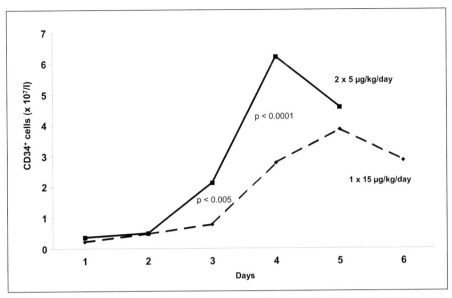

Figure 4.4-2 Increase of CD34+ cells in healthy donors after 2 x 5 μg/kg/day on days 1–3 or 1 x 15 μg/kg/day rhG-CSF on days 1–5.

Results

Donors

Administration of G-CSF and leukaphereses were completed in every donor without G-CSF dose reduction. There were few side effects during mobilization in 91 donors treated with 2 x 5 μg/kg/day G-CSF for 3 days. Moderate bone pain (WHO grade I) was observed in 25 donors. Only 3 donors developed intense bone pain (WHO grade II) and mild fever. In contrast, almost all stem cell donors treated with 1 x 15 μg/kg/day for 5 days reported some side effects due to G-CSF application. 23 donors complained of bone pain, especially back and pelvis pain (WHO grade I), and 5 complained of strong bone pain, fever or headache (WHO grade II). All stem cell donors reported that bone pain, fever and headache resolved within 3 days after termination of G-CSF application.

The number of white blood cells (WBC) increased from day 2 after G-CSF and reached a peak value on day 4 or 5 in all donors. WBC count in donors receiving 15 μg/kg/day increased from 6.7 x 10⁹/l (range: 3.2–8.6) to 39.7 x 10⁹/l (range: 25.3–73.3) while in donors receiving 5 μg/kg/12 h the total WBC count went from base-line value of 6.6 x 10⁹/l (range: 3.1–14.1) to 48.5 x 10⁹/l (range: 23.0–82.7) respectively. The WBC count was significantly higher on days 2–4 for donors receiving G-CSF twice a day in comparison to donors receiving G-CSF only once a day (Fig. 4.4-1).

CD34+ cells were mobilized with different kinetics for the two groups. The peak values of CD34+ cells in donors treated with G-CSF once a day were slower and significantly lower than those in donors treated with G-CSF twice a day on day 3 and 4 (Fig. 4.4-2). The highest value of CD34+ cells was detected

Table 4.4-2   Comparison of apheresis products between *group 1* (2 x 5 μg/kg/day) and *group 2* (1 x 15 μg/kg/day).

Group	Volume of apheresis (l)	MNC (x 10^8/kg)	CD34+ (x 10^6/kg)	CFU-GM (x 10^4/kg)	CD3+ (x 10^8/kg)
1	24.0	10.4	6.8	74.1	3.8
(range)	(15.0–51.0)	(5.1–45.3)	(2.7–32.9)	(15.4–215.3)	(1.5–21.8)
2	30.0	12.5	5.9	63.4	4.3
(range)	(15.0–70.0)	(4.3–20.3)	(3.1–16.7)	(7.1–178.3)	(1.0–11.0)
p	n.s.	n.s.	n.s.	< 0.05	n.s.

after 4 days of treatment with G-CSF in the first group, and after 5 days in the second group.

In addition, a significant rise of lymphocyte subpopulations was recognized in 17 healthy donors who received G-CSF 2 x 5 μg/kg/day: CD3+ cells from 1.54 x 10^9/l to 2.55 x 10^9/l, CD4+ cells from 0.99 x 10^9/l to 1.44 x 10^9/l and CD8+ cells from 0.50 x 10^9/l to 0.78 x 10^9/l. The effect on the subpopulations of lymphocytes disappeared directly after termination of G-CSF.

Results of leukaphereses

The aphereses were mostly very well tolerated. We collected PBPC from a 3- to 5-fold blood volume by 1 or 2 aphereses on day 3 and 4 (n = 41) or day 4 (n = 50) in the first group, and by 1–3 aphereses on day 4 (n = 14), on day 4 and 5 (n = 17), or on days 4–6 (n = 2) in the second group. The comparison between the two groups is shown in Table 4.4-2.

The average number of CD34+ cells of the graft was 6.8 x 10^6/kg body weight in the first group and 5.9 x 10^6/kg in the second group, and was generally higher than the required 4.0 x 10^6/kg. Only 4 grafts failed to reach the required number of CD34+ cells by a small amount.

Discussion

This retrospective analysis focused on the optimal administration schedule for mobilization of PBPC and timing of apheresis in normal donors for allogeneic PBPC transplantation. In agreement with a previously published study [2] with 3 different schedules of G-CSF for mobilization of PBPC in normal donors, including a single daily dose of 10 μg/kg/day for 5 days and doses of 6 or 8 μg/kg/12 h for 5 days, our results suggest that administration of G-CSF in normal donors at doses of 2 x 5 μg/kg/day mobilizes significantly more CD34+ cells than 1 x 15 μg/kg/day given in a single dose. G-CSF-induced mobilization is characterized by a significant increase in the number of PBPC starting between 2 and 3 days after initiation of G-CSF treatment and reaching an optimal level within 4 days in healthy donors who received 2 x 5 μg/kg/day and within 5 days in donors who received 1 x 15 μg/kg/day. In general, the observed side effects were acceptable.

References

1. ANDERLINI, P., *et al.*: Clinical toxicity and laboratory effects of granulocyte-colony stimulating factor (filgrastim) mobilization and blood stem cell apheresis from normal donors, and analysis of charges for the procedures. Transfusion 36 (1996) 590.

2. ARBONA, C., *et al.*: Comparison between once a day vs twice a day G-CSF for mobilization of peripheral blood progenitor cells (PBPC) in normal donors for allogeneic PBPC transplantation. Bone Marrow Transplant 22 (1998) 39.

3. CLEAVER, S.A., *et al.*: Use of G-CSF to mobilize PBSC in normal healthy donors – an international survey. Bone Marrow Transplant 21 (suppl 3) (1998) 29.

4. GRATWOHL, A., *et al.*: Blood and marrow transplantation in Europe 1995. Bone marrow Transplant 19 (1997) 407.

5. GUTENSOHN, K., *et al.*: Durchflußzytometrische Analyse CD34-exprimierender hämato-poetischer Zellen in Blut und Zytaphereseprodukten. Infusionsther Transfusionsmed 23 (suppl 2) (1996) 1.

6. DE HAAS, M., *et al.*: Granulocyte colony-stimulating factor administration to healthy volunteers: Analysis of the immediate activating effect on circulating neutrophiles. Blood 84 (1994) 3885.

7. HÖGLUND, M., *et al.*: Mobilization of CD34+ cells by glycosylated and nonglycosylated G-CSF in healthy volunteers – a comparative study. Eur J Haematol 59 (1997) 177.

8. KWANO, Y., *et al.*: Peripheral blood stem cell mobilization with granulocyte colony-stimulating factor and a harvesting procedure in pediatric donors. Bone Marrow Transplant 21 (suppl 3) (1998) 32.

9. POLLMÄCHER, T., *et al.*: Effects of granulocyte colony-stimulating factor on plasma cytokine and cytokine receptor levels and on the in vivo host response to endotoxin in healthy men. Blood 87 (1996) 900.

10. WIESNETH, M., *et al.*: Mobilization and collection of allogeneic peripheral blood progenitor cells for transplantation. Bone Marrow Transplant 21 (suppl 3) (1998) 21.

4.5 Bone Marrow Alterations Induced by High-Dose Chemotherapy prior to Transplantation with Autologous Peripheral Blood Cells

Koch[1]*, St. and W. Schultze[2]

[1] Institut für Pathologie, [2] Klinik für Innere Medizin, HUMAINE Klinikum Bad Saarow/Fürstenwalde, Ost-Brandenburgisches Tumorzentrum, Bad Saarow, Germany

* To whom correspondence should be addressed (hkbs_pathologie@t-online.de)

Summary

Morphological changes after bone marrow transplantation with peripheral blood stem cell transfusion are induced by chemotherapy and/or radiation used for conditioning in the pre-transplant period. Therefore they have many similarities to changes after chemotherapy for malignant tumours. In autologous transplantation the graft-versus-host reaction can be neglected.

Two main complexes of morphological alterations are apparent: In the earliest period, a massive damage to stroma and parenchyma prevails. The morphological characteristics are numerous, i.e., extensive necrosis, destruction of fatty tissue, stromal oedema with eosinophilic exudates, sinusoidal ectasia, slight fibrosis of reticular fibres, accumulation of haemosiderophages and, mostly, a small inflammatory reaction with lymphocytes, plasma cells and mast cells. Ordinarily, in the second week after initiation of therapy, haematopoietic regeneration takes place, as well as, usually age-related, the repopulation of bone marrow at the end of the first month. Unilinear clusters of early myeloid or erythroid cells are the first feature of haematopoietic restitution. Megakaryopoiesis is usually last to develop. The regeneration of bone marrow stroma is characterized by sealing and proliferation of sinusoidal blood vessels, by resorption of interstitial bleeding as well as eosinophilic exudate. The restitution of fatty tissue and the reduction of iron deposits completes this phase.

Introduction

High-dose chemotherapy is used as a tool for eradicating malignant tumour cell infiltrations in tissues and organs by applying cytostatics in very high doses and using dose escalation. As a consequence, complete ablation of myelopoiesis occurs. Circulating haematopoietic stem cells are then collected by subsequent leukapheresis. Haematopoietic stem cells are harvested *ex vivo* and cryopreserved, pending retransplantation immediately after administration of high-dose chemotherapy. This regimen precludes the development of GvHD [4]. Nevertheless, morphological alterations comparable to those seen in GvHD can be observed, particularly after infusion of immunocompetent cells present in non-irradiated blood products.

Bone marrow findings after high-dose chemotherapy with stem cell rescue

The normal bone marrow function rests on several structural elements, e.g., bone marrow stroma and, secondly, bone marrow parenchyma (Table 4.5-1). Cytostatic therapy as well as radiation will induce alterations of both anatomical components and consequently disturb the microenvironment.

The morphological findings are similar to changes seen after tumour chemotherapy and/or radiation [1,2,3,6,7]. The early phase is characterized by massive destruction of bone marrow stroma and bone marrow parenchyma. The following late phase shows a gradual haematopoietic regeneration. The complete recovery of both bone marrow stroma and microenvironment is a prerequisite to regeneration of haematopoiesis. The morphological changes of the early phase comprise:

• necrosis;
• destruction of fat cells;
• oedema with eosinophilic exudate;
• sinusoidal ectasia;
• haemosiderin-laden macrophages;
• moderate inflammatory reaction mobilizing mast cells, lymphocytes and pericapillary plasma cells;
• mild or moderate transient reticular fibrosis.

More rarely, the alterations seen after chemotherapy include reactive osteo-genesis, multifocal perivascular bony necrosis and formation of granulomas.

The extent of bone marrow suppression induced by chemotherapy shows significant inter-individual differences, influenced by age, nutritional status and general condition as well as the initial degree of bone marrow infiltration and bone marrow fibrosis. In contrast to former views, the morphological bone marrow changes induced by chemotherapy will persist over a prolonged period of time. The megaloblastic maturation disorders of haematopoiesis, mainly of erythropoiesis, are frequent, due to impairment of DNA synthesis as a result of cytostatic application [3].

Haematopoiesis resumes, usually, two weeks after completion of chemo-therapy. Thus, erythro- and granulopoiesis takes place in the early phase of regeneration, giving rise to monomorphic cells which will first be detected forming islets of grouped cells.

Table 4.5-1 Anatomical components of bone marrow.

Stroma	Parenchyma
Endost	Stem cells
Reticulum	Megakaryopoiesis
Vascular system	Granulocytopoiesis
Fatty tissue	Erythropoiesis
Nervous tissue	Lymphopoiesis
	Monocytes
	Plasma cells

Table 4.5-2 Sequence of haematopoietic regeneration (according to [5]).

Time after chemotherapy (days)	Morphological changes
7	Few unilinear erythropoietic und granulopoietic cell colonies, dyshaematopoietic cell alterations
7–14	Appearance of megakaryocytes
14–21	Mixed erythro- and granulocytopoietic cell islands
17	Amount of granulocytes > 0.005 gpt/l
20	Amount of leucocytes > 2 gpt/l
21	50% normal cellularity
4th week	100% normal cellularity
12th week	Normal amounts of T- and B-lymphocytes in the peripheral blood

Megakaryopoietic regeneration phenomena are visible in the late phase of reconstitution. The normal, age-related repopulation with and distribution of haematopoietic cells will be reached within two to four weeks post chemotherapy. In allogeneic stem cell transplantation, regeneration usually requires a longer period [3]. Persistent hypocellularity or cytopenia may result from impaired regeneration following viral infection. The sequence of haematopoietic regeneration is shown in Table 4.5-2.

Regeneration in bone marrow stroma is morphologically characterized by:
• sealing and proliferation of sinusoidal vessels;
• resorption of bleedings;
• gradual degradation of eosinophilic substance;
• degeneration of transient reticular fibrosis (which is often connected with an extramedullary/intrasinusoidal haematopoiesis);
• reduction of iron deposits because of iron incorporation in erythrocytes (leading to a decrease in iron-laden macrophages);
• restitution of fat cells ("clean" pattern of fatty tissue);
• consecutive hypercellularity of bone marrow under conditions of focal irradiation in nonirradiated areas with transformation of fat cells into haematopoietic tissue.

The regeneration of erythropoiesis is characterized by:
• appearance of compact islets with only small intercellulary spaces which are greater and more dense than normal erythropoietic islands;
• localization in paratrabecular and central zones;
• many cells at the same stage of maturation;
• mitosis, nuclear atypias, megaloblastic structure;
• rapid proliferation (high sensitivity to chemotherapeutic substances).

The regeneration of granulopoiesis is more resistant to chemotherapy than is erythropoiesis. The granulopoiesis shows:
• disseminated localization of the early granulopoietic cell groups in the bone marrow cavity (also in the centre of bone marrow and in the erythropoietic islands);

- low cohesiveness of the individual cells;
- varying amount of left shift.

The regeneration of megakaryopoiesis usually occurs later than the regeneration of erythro- and granulopoiesis; dysmegakaryopoiesis, however, is always decreased with anomalies of the nuclei, e.g., hypo- and hyperlobulation, bizarre forms.

Specific diagnostic problems and practical conclusions regarding morphological diagnostics

High-dose chemotherapy with autologous stem cell rescue is a useful approach in the treatment of a broad spectrum of different haematological and non-haematological neoplasias. With respect to the evaluation of cytological and histological slides of bone marrow specimens, diagnostic problems may be encountered especially with the following disease entities:
- acute leukaemia;
- myelodysplastic syndromes;
- chronic myeloproliferative syndromes, especially chronic myelocytic leukaemia;
- evaluation of residual infiltrates in acute myelocytic and lymphocytic leukaemia, and in plasmocytoma.

Using solely morphological methods, the differentiation between purely regenerative alterations and residual cells and cell groups originating from the haematological malignancy treated in the first place may be hazardous. In addition to histological and cytological findings, the clinical course and the results of immunophenotyping must be taken into account. The histological bone marrow examination is suitable especially for the investigation of stromal changes and of residual infiltrates, with immuno-histochemical methods still being a valuable contribution.

References

1. BAIN, B.J, ET AL.:H: Knochenmarkpathologie. Atlas und Lehrbuch, Blackwell Wissenschafts-Verlag, Berlin (2000) 235–238.
2. FRISCH, B. and R. BARTL: Biopsy interpretation of bone and bone marrow. London, Arnold (1999) 338–349.
3. FOUCAR, M.K.: Interpretation of Postchemotherapy and Posttransplantation Bone Marrow Specimens. In: Knowles, D.M. (Ed.), Neoplastic Haematopathology. 2nd. Ed., Philadelphia, Baltimore, New York, Lippincott, Williams & Wilkin (2001) 1791–1813.
4. OSTENDORF, P.C., U.W. SCHAEFER and A.R. ZANDER: Knochenmarktransplantation. In: P.C. Ostendorf, S. Seeber, Hämatologie, Onkologie. München, Urban & Schwarzenberg (1997) 222–236.
5. SALE, G.E. and C.D. BUCKNER: Pathology of bone marrow transplant recipients. Haematol Oncol Clin North Am 2 (1988) 735–756.
6. VAN DEN BERG, H., et al.: Early reconstitution of haemato-poiesis after allogenic bone marrow transplantation: a prospective histopathological study of bone marrow biopsy specimens. J Clin Pathol 43 (1990) 365–369.
7. WILKINS, B.S., et al.: Haematopoietic regrowth after chemotherapy for acute leukaemia: an immunohistochemical study of bone marrow trephine biopsy specimens. J Clin Pathol 46 (1993) 915–921.

4.6 Susceptibility Testing of Pathogenic Yeasts Causing Systemic Mycoses

Czaika[1]*, V. A., A. F. Schmalreck[2], H.-J. Tietz[3], S. Koch[1], G. K. Czaika[4], M. Ossadnik[1], W. Sterry[3], W. Schultze[1]

[1] HUMAINE-Klinikum Bad Saarow, Dept. of Internal Medicine (Affiliation: Charité University Hospital, Berlin) and Ostbrandenburgisches Tumorzentrum, [2] Microbiological Service Munich, Munich, [3] Universitätshautklinik der Charité, Berlin, [4] DRK-Kliniken Westend, Dept. of Internal Medicine, Berlin, Germany

* To whom correspondence should be addressed

Introduction and Results

Primary and secondary fungal infections are among the most frequent infections, ranking fourth in intensive care units in the US, for instance, with a tendency to increasing incidence world-wide. Considering this status and the introduction of several new anti-fungal agents, antifungal susceptibility testing is required (i) in order to detect yeast spread and resistant strains, for purely epidemiological purposes, and (ii) for the evaluation of susceptibility patterns and, in addition, the selection of the appropriate antifungal agent. Furthermore, with agents like fluconazole, which will increase blood and/or tissue levels with increasing dose, quantitative susceptibility testing of the pathogen is a prerequisite with respect to best therapeutic effects. At present, standardized testing methods fulfilling these requirements are in practice in the USA (NCCLS, M27 A) and Germany (DIN 58940-84). Moreover, the NCCLS introduced the assessment category DD, i.e. dose-dependent susceptibility, to cover those pathogenic yeasts possessing higher minimum inhibitory concentrations (MIC), and thus requiring higher doses as a prerequisite to successful therapy.

Susceptibility Testing

Susceptibility testing was performed by microdilution with YST medium according to DIN 58940-84. Susceptibility rates for fluconazole and *C. albicans* were determined as 97% (n = 1398; mode MIC, 1.0 mg/l), *C. glabrata* 87% (n = 312; 4.0), *C. guilliermondii* 32% (n = 88; 32.0), *C. kefyr* 100% (n = 27; 1.0), *C. krusei* 43% (n = 180; 32.0), *C. lusitaniae* 93% (n = 40; 2.0), *C. parapsilosis* 94% (n = 137; 0.13), *Cryptococcus neoformans* 75% (n = 132; 4.0), *Exophiala dermatitidis* 84% (n = 64; 4.0). The overall rate of resistant isolates for all yeast strains tested (n = 2776) were for amphotericin B: 3%, fluconazole 11%, flucytosine 7%, itraconazole 13%, ketoconazole 7%, voriconazole 4% and terbinafine (n = 127) 74%. Fluconazole, because of the good tolerance and the high doses which can be administered (approx. 12 mg/kg, in one report even up to 30 mg/kg), is a very widely used anti-fungal agent and one of the first-line drugs, particularly in the treatment of infections by *Candida* spp., except for *C. krusei* and sometimes *C. glabrata*, *C. guilliermondii* and *C. tropicalis* isolates.

Conclusion

In spite of the general use, and despite some reports about acquired resistance in isolates from HIV patients under continuous treatment, there has been no decrease in fluconazole susceptibility, comparing the testing periods of 1993/1994 and 1998/99, with respect to the pathogens covered. In the present context, it should be added that fluconazole is also commonly used as prophylaxis in transplant patients.

References

1. DENNING, D., *et al.*: Azole resistance in *Candida*. Eur J Clin Microbiol Infect Dis 4 (1997) 261–280.
2. E DIN 58940-84 Medizinische Mikrobiologie – Empfindlichkeitsprüfung von mikrobiellen Krankheitserregern gegen Chemotherapeutika – Teil 84. Mikrodilution – Spezielle Anforderungen an die Testung von Pilzen gegen Antimykotika. Deutsches Institut für Normung, Beuth Verlag Berlin (1999).
3. ESPINEL-INGROFF, A.: Antifungal Susceptibility Testing. Clin Microbiol Newslett 18 (1996) 161–166.
4. FORTÚN, J., *et al.*: Selection of *Candida glabrata* Strains with Reduced Susceptibility to Azoles in Four Liver Transplant Patients with Invasive Candidiasis. Eur J Clin Microbiol 16 (1997) 314–318.
5. FRITSCH, P.: (1998) Pilzkrankheiten (Mykosen) In: Dermatology and Venerologie: Lehrbuch und Atlas. Springer Verlag Berlin, Heidelberg, New York, 289–295.
6. KUNZELMANN, V., *et al.*: Voraussetzungen für eine effektive Therapie chronisch rezidivierender Vaginalcandidosen. Mycoses 39 (Suppl. 1) (1996) 65–72.
7. MORSCHHÄUSER, J., *et al.*: Virulenz- und Resistenzmechanismen pathogener *Candida* Spezies. Med. Welt 48 (1997) 352–357.
8. NATIONAL COMMITTEE FOR CLINICAL LABORATORY STANDARDS: Reference method for broth dilution antifungal susceptibility testing of yeasts. Approved standard. M27. National Committee for Clinical Laboratory Standards. Wayne, Philadelphia (1998).
9. NOLTING, S., *et al.*: Terbinafine in onchomycosis with involvment by non-dermatophytic fungi. Br J Dermatol (Suppl.) 43 (199) 16–21.
10. PETRANYI, G. , *et al.*: Antifungal activity of the allylamine derivate terbinafine *in vitro*. Antimcrob Ag Chemother 31 (199) 1365–1368.
11. PITROW, L. and PENK, A. : Plasma und Gewebekonzentrationen von Fluconazol: Diskussion der Breakpoint-Problematik. Mycoses 39 (Suppl. 2) (1996) 58–65.
12. REX, J.H.: Resistance of *Candida* Species to Fluconazole. Antimicrob Ag Chemother 39 (1995) 1–8.
13. RYDER S.R. and B. Favre: Antifungal Activity and Mechanism of Action of Terbinafin. Contemp Pharmacother. 8 (1997) 275–287.
14. SCHMALRECK, A.F., *et al.*: An evaluation of seven methods of testing *in vitro* susceptibility of clinical yeast isolates to fluconazole. Mycoses 38 (1995) 359–368.
15. SCHMALRECK, A.F., *et al.*: Differentiation and characterisation of yeasts (*Candida albicans*, *Exophiala dermatitidis*) and animal pathogen algae (*Prototheca* spp.) by Fourier Transform Infrared Spectroscopy (FT-IR) in comparison to conventional methods. Mycoses 41 (1998) 71–77.
16. SOBEL, J. D.: Vulvovaginitis due to *Candida glabrata*. An emerging problem. Mycoses 41 (Suppl. 2) (1998) 18–22.
17. TIETZ, H.J., *et al.*: Case Report. Osteomyelitis caused by high resistant *Candida guilliermondii*. Mycoses 42 (1999) 577–580.
18. VAN'T WOUT, J.W.: Fluconazole treatment of *Candida* infections caused by non-*albicans* *Candida* species. Eur J Clin Microbiol Infect Dis 15 (1996) 238–243.

19. VUFFRAY, A., *et al.*: Oropharyngeal candidiasis resistant to single-dose therapy with fluconazole in HIV-infected patients. AIDS 8 (1994) 708–709.
20. WEBB, D.: New Antifungal Agents: Clinical and Laboratory Issues. Clin Microbiol Newslett 13 (1991) 129–133.
21. WILDFEUER, A.: Fluconazole: comparison of pharmacokinetics, therapy and *in vitro* susceptibility. Mycoses 40 (1997) 259–265.
22. WILDFEUER, A., *et al.*: Fluconazole: comparison of pharmacokinetics, therapy and *in vitro* susceptibility. Mycoses 40 (1997) 259–265.

4.7 Radical *in vivo* Elimination of Dysregulated T-Cells and/or Hyperactivated Accessory Cells on the Humoral plus Cellular Level. Results in the Pre-Disease State. Graft-versus-Malignancy (GvM) Effect as a Special Case of this Strategy

Leskovar *, P. and R. Schmidmaier

Immunological-Biochemical Research Laboratory, Dept. of Urology, Medical School, Technical University, Munich, Germany

* To whom correspondence should be addressed (peter@leskovar.de)

Introduction

Various diseases are characterized by an overstimulation of antigen specific and non-specific T-cell subsets which are in a permanent intimate contact with (over)stimulated accessory cells. This hyperactivation of disease-related subsets is accompanied by an increased plasma level of some surface structures shed from the hyperactivated immunocytes. Interestingly, these solubilized membrane molecules are identical, independent of the kind and type of the underlying disorder.

Clinical observations show indeed that diseases as different as (advanced) cancer, chronic bacterial and (retro)viral infections (including HIV) and granulomatous inflammations (sarcoidosis, CGD) are associated with increased levels of the same hyperactivity markers, such as β2-microglobulin (β2m), whose plasma level is increased in multiple myeloma [5], lymphoma [3], CLL [19], further in autoimmune disorders such as SLE [18] or rheumatoid arthritis [17] and in viral infections, e.g. EBV [16], hepatitis B [6] and HIV [7]. The β2m plasma level is also increased in recipients of renal transplants [20]. Neopterin is a further example of hyperactivation markers, shared by the broad spectrum of the above mentioned disorders. They cannot, however, be discussed here. Though AIDS is characterized by severe immune suppression, both the percentage of activated, MHC II-expressing T-cells and the plasma concentration of different markers of immunocyte hyperactivation, such as neopterin/monopterin [2], lysozyme [3], sCD8 [13] and acid-labile alpha-interferon [1], in addition to the above-mentioned β2m, are significantly increased in HIV-infected persons. Resting cells are normally MHC II-negative, except for a low percentage of cells with suppressive properties. The activated state, in turn, is associated with the coexpression of the class II-antigens [14,15]. These phenomena have been studied in the allogeneic system [8] and during T-cell activation by soluble antigens [11] when first T4 and then T8 cells become MHC II-positive. Cancer, chronic infections and AIDS are associated with the high percentage of HLA-DR and CD8-positive T-lymphocytes. It seems that these T-cells are active suppressor cells ("effector Ts cells"), since a persistent stimulation of T-cells results in a selective generation of the Ts subset [4]. In spite of the clonotypic diversity, the pathologically dysregulated T-cells in different disorders often belong to the same basic T-cell subset.

Conclusions

The GvM effect can be considered as a special case of a more general phenomenon that could be described as "graft-versus-dysregulated-immuno-cytes" effect and may work in all diseases, which are characterized by a hyperactivated or persistently (over)stimulated state of immunocompetent cells, primarily the T-cells and/or accessory cells. The novel therapeutic principle is based on the *in vivo* depletion of these dysregulated, disease-inducing and maintaining immunocyte subsets whose common vulnerable site are (hyper)activation-associated membrane structures, such as MHC II. If these pathological T-cell (and APC) subsets are radically eliminated on the humoral plus cellular level, the pre-disease state can be re-established, as shown in the murine B16 melanoma model for neoplastic diseases and in two rat models for autoimmune disorders, i.e. the adjuvant arthritis (AA) and the experimental allergic encephalomyelitis (EAE) model.

The crucial cellular component of this radical *in vivo* elimination of dysregulated immunocytes is provided by the novel MIS ("microimmuno-surgery") and MIT ("microimmunotargeting") effectors which recognize the above mentioned (hyper)activation membrane structures. The immuno-intervention by these donor-derived effector cells is time-limited, due to their pre-programmed cell death. The eliminated, pathologically dysregulated immunocyte subsets are later completely replaced by post-recruited naive subclones.

In the animal model, we were able to confirm the high therapeutical efficacy of the novel MIS/MIT approach in all systems tested until now, i.e. the cancer, the autoimmune and the transplantation (GvH/HvG) models. The 100% long-term survival of mice whose tumour-protecting suppressor T-cells (not tumour cells *per se*) have been radically depleted by the MIS/MIT treatment strongly supports the idea of cancer as an immunoregulatory problem rather than an irreversible end-state.

References

1. ABB, J., F. DEINHARDT: Human interferon-alpha production in homosexual men with AIDS. J Infect Dis 150(1) (1984) 158.
2. ABITA, J. P.: Urinary neopterin and biopterin levels in patients with AIDS and ARC. Lancet 6 (1985)51.
3. AMLOT, P. L., M. ADINOLFI: Serum β2-microglobulin and ist prognostic value in lymphomas. Eur J Cancer 15 (1979) 79.
4. AUNE, I.M., S.L. POGUE: Generation and characterization of continuous line of CD8+ suppressor T-lympholcytes. J Immunol 142 (11) (1989) 3731.
5. BATAILLE, R., J. GRENIER: β2-Microglobulin in multiple myeloma. Optimal use for staging prognosis and treatment. A prospective study of 160 patients. Blood 63 (1984) 468.
6. BEORCHIA, et al.: Elevation of serum β2-microglobulin in liver diseases. Clin Chim Acta 109(1981) 245.
7. BHALLA, R.B., et al.: Abnormally high concentrations of β2-microglobulin in AIDS patients. Clin Chem 29 (1983) 1560.
8. BRODSKY, F.M., et al.: Monoclonal antibodies to HLA-DRw determinants. Tissue Antigens 16 (1980) 30.

9. BROWN, M.F., *et al.:* Cloned human T-cells synthesize Ia molecules and can function as APCs. Hum Immunol 11 (1984) 219.

10. ENGELMAN, E.G., *et al.:* Leukocytes in man. II; Functional studies of HLA-DR positive cells activated in MLC. J Exp Med 152 (1980) 114.

11. FAINBOIM, L., *et al.:* Precursor and effector phenotypes of activated human T-lymphocytes. Nature 288 (1980) 391.

12. FESTENSTEIN, H., *et al.:* Changing antigenic profiles of HLA class II antigens on activated T-cells and their biological effects. In: HLA class II antigens (Ed. Solheim, B.G., Moeller, E.C., Ferrone, S.), Springer/Berlin-N.Y. (1986) 314–338.

13. FUCHS, D., *et al.:* Immunaktivierungsmarker zur Verlaufskontrolle der HIV-Infektion, Symposium-Volume, München AIDS Tage, Jan. 19–21 (1990).

14. GREAVES, M. F., *et al.:* Ia-like antigens on human T-cells. Eur J Immunol 9 (1979) 356.

15. KO, H.S., *et al.:* Ia determinants on stimulated human T-lymphocytes. Occurrence on mitogen and antigen activated T-cells. J Exp Med 180 (1979) 246.

16. LAMELIN, J. P., *et al.:* Elevation of serum β2-microglobulin levels during infectious mononucleosis. Clin Immunol Immunopathol 24 (1982) 55.

17. REVILLARD C., *et al.:* β2-microglobulin and β2-microglobulin-binding proteins in inflammatory diseases. Eur J Rheumatol Inflam 5 (1982) 398.

18. REVILLARD C., *et al.:* Anti-β2-microglobulin cytotoxic antibodies in systemic lupus erythematosus. J Immunol 122 (1979) 614.

19. SIMONSSON, S., *et al.:* β2-microglobulin in chronic lymphocytic leukemia. Scand J Haematol 24 (1980) 174.

20. VINCENT, C., *et al.:* β2-microglobulin in monitoring renal transplant function. Transplant Proc 11(1979) 438.

4.8 Discrimination between T-Cell Subsets Involved in GvM and GvH Effects, respectively, and the Resulting Therapeutic Consequences

Leskovar *, P. and R. Schmidmaier

Immunological-Biochemical Research Laboratory, Dept. of Urology, Medical School, Technical University, Munich, Germany

* To whom correspondence should be addressed (peter@leskovar.de)

Summary

We show for the first time that the beneficial, strongly tumouricidal graft-versus-malignancy (GvM) effect can be separated from the adverse graft-versus-host (GvH) side effect, as both are caused, at least partly, by T-cell clones, differing both in their clonotypic specificity and origin. The GvM effect, which comprises the graft-versus-leukaemia (GvL) and the graft-versus-tumour (GvT) effect, represents one of the strongest anti-tumour reactions; it is, however, associated with a high risk of the potentially fatal GvHD. Therefore, the mentioned dissection of the involved T-cell clones opens new avenues in the selective enhancement of the curative GvM effect, without a parallel induction of the adverse GvHD side effect.

The antitumour effect of allogeneic donor cells, termed graft-versus-malignancy(GvM)-effect, which can be observed in recipients of allogeneic bone marrow or stem cell grafts [2,5,10] and in patients with BMT relapse, treated by donor lymphocytes (DLs) [1,6,7], is generally accepted.

Is the discrimination between the GvM and GvH reaction possible?

The GvM effect, which can be subdivided into the GvL and the GvT effect, appears to be a complex immune reaction, implicating immunocompetent cells (T-cells, APCs/macrophages) of both donor and host origin. The GvHR, on the contrary, seems to include only donor-derived immunocytes. The evaluation of our animal experiments led to the conclusion that the GvM effect is caused by two separate T-cell subsets, differing in their origin and in their specificity. The first subset, responsible for the GvM/I sub-effect, seems to be of donor origin and represents the recipient-specific alloreactive T-cells. It is undistinguishable from the GvHD-inducing T-cell subset. The second subset, responsible for the GvM/II sub-effect, seems to be host-derived and consists of deblocked, tumour-specific cytotoxic T-cells (Tc/CTLs), enriched with host's post-recruited tumouricidal CTLs; this subset is unique for the GvM effect and does not play any role in the GvHD complication. The GvM/II effect, however, substantially depends on the GvM/I effect because the deblocking of pre-existing tumour-specific CTLs – as prerequisite for the GvM/II sub-effect – results from the GvM/I-mediated *in vivo* inactivation of tumour-specific suppressor T-cells (Ts). These tumour-protecting Ts cells represent the preferential targets of GvM/I-effectors due to their coexpression of class-II-MHC antigens, since the alloreactive GvM/I-effectors show no preference for malignant versus nonmalignant cells but rather for class-II-MHC-coexpressing vs. MHC II-negative targets.

As deduced from cellular HLA-typing techniques such as primary and secondary MLC, CML and PLT, the direct targets of donor effector cells appear to be the MHC II-expressing T-cells, in addition to the MHC II-positive monocytes/macrophages and/or B cells [3,4,8]. When histoincompatible lymphocytes from person A and person B are coincubated in the one-way MLC, alloreactive CTLs are generated only if A and B show both the class-I- and the class-II-MHC incompatibility. In the case that the incompatibility is restricted to the MHC I complex, no cell proliferation (MLC test) and no alloreactive CTLs (CML test) are generated. If, on the other hand, the MHC mismatch is restricted to the class-II antigens, only Th-proliferation but no CTL-generation is observed [3,4,8]. The critical event for the activation and clonal expansion of alloreactive CTLs seems to be the cooperation of their precursors (pCTLs) with (primed or non-primed) Th cells on the surface of APCs or other MHC-II-coexpressing cells. If T-cells are activated by alloantigens, the Th and the Tc cells do not belong to the same subpopulation, expressing the same T-cells receptor, since the Th cells recognize the class-II incompatibility ("altered-self"-/"non-self"-MHC II) and the CTLs (pCTLs) the class-I-incompatible structures ("altered-self"-/"non-self"-MHC I) which are normally not identical [3,4,8]. It seems that good Th and Tc cooperation is possible even between T subpopulations with differing antigenic specificities. More important than a TCR identity appears to be the coexpression of class-II- and class-I-MHC antigens on the surface of (autologous or allogeneic) APC, or on the surface of MHC I and MHC II double positive (allogeneic) target cell; in other terms, the generation of both the alloreactive Tc cells and the allospecific Th cells requires the expression of the MHC II-complex in addition to the MHC I-antigens on the stimulating target cells. Due to the local stimulation of CTLs by costimulated helper T-cells (Th), they show, as discussed above, preference rather for MHC II-coexpressing targets than for malignant cells.

Once deblocked, tumour-specific CTLs exert their tumouricidal effect as so-called GvM/II-effectors, whereas the allospecific GvM/I-effectors seem to play rather an indirect, immunoregulatory role by inactivating tumour-protecting Ts/Th2 cells. There is, however, a mutual interdependence of the two GvM sub-effects because the donor-derived GvM/I-effectors must first be *in vivo* (or *in vitro*) allopreimmunized by the host's APCs. This effect could explain the significantly better results in CML patients than in ALL patients treated by DLI for BMT relapse [7]. In ALL patients, the myeloablative preconditioning of marrow graft recipients also critically reduced the patient's APCs, necessary for the activation of GvM/I-effectors, a problem being circumvented in CML patients by the MHC II-coexpression on malignant targets and a higher number of APC-mimicking residual CML cells. Since the pioneering experiments of A. SINGER, R. ZINKERNAGEL, A. ALTHAGE and colleagues in the early 1980s [9, 11, 12] we know that the fine structural differences between transformed and normal cells, i.e. the tumour-specific antigens (TSA), can be recognized solely by autologous and – in the animal model – syngeneic T-cells, showing the MHC restriction for tumour targets. So the special role of donor-derived effectors is not the recognition and killing of tumour cells *per se* but rather the deblockade and post-recruitment of the patient's own tumour-specific CTLs. The fact that in haematologic malignancies, in contrast to the situation in solid tumours, the direct alloaggressive action of the GvM/I-effectors is able to coeradicate malignant cells can be explained by the easy access, often associated with the MHC II coexpression, in haematologic malignancies in contrast to the situation in solid tumours. In solid tumours, this direct tumouricidal effect of GvM/I-effectors, based on the MHC-mismatch rather than on tumour-specific structures of malignant targets, is negligible, so that the antitumour activity of GvM/I-effectors is indirect, i.e. rather regulatory. The recent trend in allogeneic HSCT to replace myeloablative preconditioning by the immunoablative one [1,6,7] mediately underlines the importance of the GvM/II effect in the prevention of tumour relapses.

Novel strategy, based on the GvHD-free GvL effect

Our novel strategy, called "microimmunosurgery" (MIS), is based on a strong GvM effect without the risk of the GvHD side effect. The selective, MIS-mediated GvM effect is the result of the *in vitro* premanipulation of MIS effectors by a multistep procedure, conferring on the engineered effector cells (a) pre-programmed lifespan (with the preceding step of cell cycle-synchronization), (b) increased cytolytic capacity, (c) resistance against hyperpolarization-induced anergy, and (d) partial Th1-type reprogramming of host's (patient's) accessory cells.

References

1. FRASSONI, F., *et al.*: The effect of donor leukocyte infusion in patients with leukemia following allogeneic bone marrow transplantation. Exp Hematol 20 (1992) 712.
2. GIRALT, S. A., R.E. CHAMPLIN: Leukemia relapse after allogeneic bone marrow transplantation. A review. Blood 84 (1994) 3603.
3. HARDY, D. A., *et al.*: Destruction of lymphoid cells by activated human lymphocytes. Nature 227 (1970) 723.
4. HARMON, W. E., *et al.*: Comparison of cell-mediated lympholysis and mixed lymphocyte culture in the immunologic evaluation for renal transplantation. J Immunol 129(1982)1573.
5. HOROWITZ, M. M., *et al.*: Graft-versus-leukemia reactions after bone marrow transplantation. Blood 75 (1990) 555.
6. KOLB, H. J., *et al.*: Donor leukocyte transfusions for treatment of recurrent chronic myelogenous leukemia in marrow transplant patients. Blood 76 (1990) 2462.
7. KOLB, H. J., *et al.*: Graft-versus-leukemia effect of donor lymphocyte transfusions in marrow grafted patient. Blood 86/5 (11995) 2041.
8. KRISTENSEN, T.: Human histocompatibility testing by T-cell-mediated lympholysis: a European standard CML technique. Tissue Antigens 16 (1980) 335.
9. SINGER, A., *et al.*: Self-recognition in allogeneic radiation bone marrow chimeras. J Exp Med 153 (1981) 1286.
10. WEIDEN, P. L., *et al.*: The Seattle Marrow Transplant Team: Antileukemic effect of chronic graft-versus-host disease. Contribution to improved survival after allogeneic marrow transplantation. N Engl J Med 304 (1981) 1529.
11. ZINKERNAGEL, R. M., *et al.*: Restriction specificities, alloreactivity, and allotolerance expressed by T cells from nude mice reconstituted with H-2-compatible or -incompatible thymus graft. J Exp Med 151 (1980) 376.
12. ZINKERNAGEL, R. M., *et al.*: On the thymus in the differentiation of "H-2 self-recognition" by T cells: Evidence for dual recognition? J Exp Med 147(1978) 882.

Part Five
Solid Tumours

5.1 High-Dose Chemotherapy-Studies in Ovarian Cancer – An Overview

Wandt*, H., K. Schäfer-Eckart, W. M. Gallmeier

BMT-Unit, Klinikum Nürnberg, Germany

* To whom correspondence should be addressed (wandt@klinikum-nuernberg.de)

Summary

High-dose chemotherapy, supported by stem cell transplantation in optimally debulked patients with advanced ovarian cancer FIGO stage III and IV, yields a long-term disease-free probability of about 30%. This is a promising result, but the true value of high-dose chemotherapy has to be proven by prospective randomized trials which compare this approach to the best conventional chemotherapy. Performing high-dose chemotherapy in optimally debulked patients should be restricted to randomized studies. In suboptimally debulked patients, long-term results are disappointing, even with sequential high-dose chemotherapy. For these patients, new treatment strategies like neo-adjuvant chemotherapy followed by interval debulking and the introduction of new drugs as well as immunotherapeutic strategies are necessary.

Introduction

Patients with advanced ovarian cancer still have a poor prognosis, despite the fact that elaborated combination chemotherapies achieve response rates between 60% and 80%. Long-term disease control occurs (i) in 20% to 30% of women with optimally debulked stage III disease, (ii) in less than 10% of women with incompletely resected stage III disease, and (iii) in less than 5% of women with stage IV disease [3]. These disappointing long-term results are nearly unchanged, in spite of the introduction of paclitaxel in the conventional treatment of ovarian cancer. In order to overcome drug resistance to conventional chemotherapy, high-dose chemotherapy supported by bone marrow transplantation was first used to treat advanced ovarian cancer about 15 years ago.

Phase I/II Studies (1985–1995)

Numerous phase I/II studies have been performed worldwide in order to explore the most effective high-dose regimen with tolerable toxicity. High-dose carboplatin and alkylating agents, like cyclophosphamide and melphalan, were mostly used, and have shown high remission rates of up to 90% and 100%, with complete remission rates of up to 50% [5]. High-dose chemotherapy was used as consolidation after 4–6 cycles of conventional chemotherapy. Disease-free survival rates and overall survival of 27% and 71% respectively were reported at 5 years [2]. With the availability of peripheral blood stem cells, multiple sequential cycles of high-dose chemotherapy as first-line treatment could be applied with promising results [7]. In a US meta-analysis of such phase I/II studies, P. J. STIFF *et al.* concluded that high-dose chemotherapy should be used in optimally debulked patients with platin-sensitive tumors. Phase III trials are needed to compare these findings to those of conventional chemotherapy [4,6].

Phase III Studies (1995 – ongoing)

Based on the experiences of phase I/II studies, prospective comparative randomized trials were initiated in several countries in Europe and the US when high-dose chemotherapy and stem cell transplantation were increasingly used in breast and ovarian cancer in the mid-nineties. Following the presentation of the first negative results in high-dose chemotherapy in breast cancer at the ASCO meeting, 1999, and in connection with the Bezwoda story, gynaecologists all over the world were reluctant to offer their patients high-dose chemotherapy with stem cell support. This is the background which explains the difficulties in recruiting patients for phase III trials. As a consequence, the GOG in the United States stopped all high-dose phase III trials in ovarian cancer. The same happened with the Finland phase III study which was terminated early without a scientific result, due to poor recruitment. The French GINECO study is now finished, with 110 patients. After 3–4 cycles of conventional chemotherapy patients with documented response were randomized to either three cycles of conventional carboplatin/cyclophosphamide or one high-dose chemotherapy cycle of carboplatin (1600 mg/m^2) and cyclophosphamide (6 g/m^2). At the ASCO meeting in 2001 first results were presented, showing a significant benefit (p = 0.03) for disease-free survival in the high-dose arm [4].

Actually, there are still two ongoing phase III studies in Europe comparing sequential high-dose chemotherapy with conventional chemotherapy in advanced ovarian cancer. These are the European EBMT-OVCAT study and the German AGO/AIO study (HD-OVAR-2). Both trials compare rather well; patients up to 65 years and eligible for high-dose chemotherapy are randomized, being subjected to either 6 cycles of conventional chemotherapy (cisplatin or carboplatin plus paclitaxel; additional antracyclin is optional) or to sequential high-dose chemotherapy. Sequential high-dose chemotherapy consists of two intermediate dose cycles of cyclophosphamide (3 g/m^2) and paclitaxel (200 and 250 mg/m^2 in the EMBT and German trial, respectively). During these two cycles, G-CSF mobilized peripheral blood stem cells are collected to support the subsequent three high-dose cycles. The first two high-dose cycles are performed each with carboplatin AUC 20 and paclitaxel in the same dose as before. The third and last high-dose cycle includes melphalan 140 mg/m^2 and high-dose carboplatin AUC 20. Because paclitaxel is also used for the last high-dose cycle in the EBMT study, the total dose of paclitaxel (1000 mg/m^2) remains identical in both studies, i.e. the EBMT- and the AGO/AIO trial.

To assess whether progression-free survival at 2 and 3 years may prove statistically significant, a number of about 250 patients ought to be recruited in both studies. During the last 3 years, however, only 112 patients have been recruited. High-dose chemotherapy was well tolerated and could be performed partially on an outpatient basis. Up to now no treatment-related mortality has been observed.

Perspectives

At present, the question as to the validity of high-dose chemotherapy in ovarian cancer can, therefore, only be answered by combining the data collected in both, the EBMT- and the AGO/AIO study. The two study groups have now decided to join forces and to proceed as an intergroup trial, thus hoping for a valid answer in the near future. The recruitment pace may well increase once the first data of the GINECO study, showing a benefit for high-dose chemotherapy, has been presented at the ASCO meeting in 2001. GINECO is expected to decide soon whether or not to join the newly constituted intergroup trial.

For suboptimally debulked patients (residual tumour > 2 cm) or for patients who cannot primarily be resected, new strategies with neo-adjuvant chemotherapy and interval debulking surgery should be applied. New agents like topotecan, gemcitabine and high-dose treosulfan have to be explored. After maximal tumour debulking, gained by a combination of chemotherapy and surgery, additional immunotherapeutic strategies may be explored, for instance dendritic cell vaccination or treatment with monoclonal antibodies against epidermal growth factor.

In our Nuremberg centre, we started a "neo-adjuvant" sequential high-dose chemotherapy trial involving inoperable patients or patients who could not be optimally resected. High-dose chemotherapy consists of carboplatin, treosulfan and topotecan. The aim of the study is to maximally reduce the tumour load by sequential high-dose chemotherapy, in order to achieve a rate of 50%, or more, of patients with complete tumour resection after radical surgery. Subsequently, patients will receive an additional, weekly chemotherapy using paclitaxel, which may develop anti-angiogenic activity further to its cytotoxic action.

References

1. CURE, H., et al.: Phase III randomized trial of high-dose chemotherapy (HDC) and peripheral blood stem cell (PBSC) support as consolidation in patients (pts) with responsive low-burden advanced ovarian cancer (AOC): preliminary results of a GINECO / FNCLCC / SFGM-TC Study. ASCO 20 (2001) 815a.
2. LEGROS, M., et al.: High-dose chemotherapy with hematopoietic rescue in patients with stage III to IV ovarian cancer : long-term results. J Clin Oncol 15 (1997) 1302.
3. OMURA, G.A., et al.: Long-term follow-up and prognostic factor analysis in advanced ovarian carcinoma: the gynecologic oncology group experience. J Clin Oncol 9 (1991) 1138.
4. PATRICK, J., et al.: High-dose chemotherapy and autologous stem-cell transplantation for ovarian cancer: an autologous blood and marrow transplant registry report. American College of Physicians–American Society of Internal Medicine 501 (2000).
5. SCHILDER, R.J., et al.: Multiple cycles of high-dose chemotherapy for ovarian cancer. Sem Onc 25 (1998) 3:349.
6. STIFF, P.J., et al.: High-dose chemotherapy with autologous transplantation for persistent/ relapsed ovarian cancer : a multivariate analysis of survival for 100 consecutively treated patients. J Clin Oncol 15 (1997) 1309.

7. WANDT, H., *et al.*: Sequential cycles of high-dose chemotherapy with dose escalation of carboplatin with or without paclitaxel supported by G-CSF mobilized peripheral blood progenitor cells: a phase I/II study in advanced ovarian cancer. Bone Marrow Transpl 23 (1999) 763.

5.2 Phenotype and Kinetics of Disseminated Breast Cancer Cells

Krüger[1,5*], W. H., N. Kröger[1], F. Tögel[1], H. Renges[1], A. Badbaran[1], R. Hornung[1], R. Jung[2], K. Gutensohn[3], F. Gieseking[4], F. Jänicke[4], A. R. Zander[1]

[1] Bone Marrow Transplantation Centre, [2] Dept. of Clinical Chemistry, [3] Dept. of Transfusion Medicine, [4] Dept. of Gynaecology and Obstetrics, Eppendorf University Hospital, Hamburg, [5] Internal Medicine IV (Haematology/Oncology), Martin Luther University, Halle-Wittenberg, Halle/S., Germany

* To whom correspondence should be addressed (william.krueger@medizin.uni-halle.de)

Summary

Tumour cell contamination of stem cell collections (PSC) harvested from breast cancer patients is frequent but with findings that vary among reports. Although so-called co-mobilization of tumour cells has been hypothesized, the origin of tumour cell contamination in PSC is still unknown. A total of 47 G-CSF-mobilized PSC grafts from patients with nodal-positive (n = 30), chemosensitive metastatic (n = 11), and five women with inflammatory breast cancer were evaluated for tumour cells by immunocytochemistry. Additionally, 40 bone marrow aspirations and 23 peripheral blood samples collected prior to apheresis and after one to two cycles of conventional chemotherapy were available for examination. Tumour cell contamination of PSC correlated best with pre-harvest peripheral blood state. This was valid when the nominal (positive/negative) presence of tumour cells in peripheral blood was compared to the nominal presence of tumour cells in PSC, and when it was correlated to the tumour cell load of PSC samples (tumour cell load = tumour cells per 10^6 nucleated cells investigated). The correlation between peripheral blood and PSC was better than that between bone marrow and PSC, despite the larger sample size of bone marrow aspirations. The presence or absence of tumour cells in PSC could not be safely predicted by the presence or absence of tumour cells in bone marrow or peripheral blood alone. Diagnostic specificity seems to improve from a combination of results. No correlation was found in quantitative analysis of tumour cell contamination between bone marrow and peripheral blood. 194 data sets consisting of bone marrow and peripheral blood samples obtained prior to and after HDT, and of aliquots of PSC products, were searched with immunochemistry and rtPCR technique for disseminated tumour cells. The presence of tumour cells in bone marrow is frequent prior to and after HDT, but HDT reduces the number of tumour cells in bone marrow significantly. In contrast, there was no effect on the number of circulating tumour cells. Reinfusion of contaminated PSC products was surprisingly associated with a low number of malignant cells in bone marrow after high-dose therapy and vice versa. Disseminated cancer cells from bone marrow, peripheral blood, and PSC have been investigated by double-stain technique for uPA-R expressing cytokeratin-positive cells. uPA-R+/CK+ cells could be found in all qualities of samples, but significantly less in PSC compared to samples of other provenance ($p = 0.02$). In conclusion, the results suggest that peripheral blood and bone marrow represent different compartments for tumour cells and that contaminating tumour cells in PSC may be derived from the blood and/or marrow compartment. The tumour cell contamination of PSC cannot be safely predicted by a preceding peripheral blood or bone marrow analysis. HDT leads to a significant but not complete eradication of disseminated tumour cells. Populations of disseminated tumour cells are phenotypically heterogeneous. Epithelial cells of malignant phenotype occur in peripheral blood, bone marrow and PSC of breast cancer patients. Reduced uPA-R expression on tumour cells from leukapheresis samples may suggest a less aggressive nature of these cells compared to disseminated cells found in bone tumour cells. Furthermore, the data suggest that the phenotype of tumour cell contamination in leukapheresis products differs significantly from those of disseminated cancer cells in bone marrow or blood.

Introduction

The presence of occult disseminated tumour cells in bone marrow at the time of diagnosis worsens the prognosis of these women significantly, as compared to patients with tumour-cell negative marrows [8].

Evidently, heterogeneity of micrometastatic cancer cells in bone marrow was shown for expression of several markers [23]. Several characteristic phenotypes, such as expression of oncogenes, growth-factor receptors and others, have been associated with the process of metastasis [10]. Therefore, the phenotypical characterization of disseminated epithelial cancer cells may be an alternative approach to investigating their metastatic capacity. In breast cancer, the expression of the urokinase-like plasminogen activator receptor plays a central role in invasion and migration [28]. The expression of uPA-R on disseminated cells derived from gastric cancer has been shown in a recent investigation [1]. The first part of this study investigates the expression of the uPA-R on disseminated breast cancer cells detected in bone marrow, blood, and as tumour cell contamination in G-CSF-mobilized peripheral stem cells.

A recent study has shown that standard-dose chemotherapy can reduce micrometastatic breast cancer cells in bone marrow, but does not have the power to eliminate them completely [3]. High-dose therapy with peripheral stem cell support is a promising approach for the treatment of women with high-risk breast cancer and for the eradication of minimal residual disease [24]. An important issue in this context is the presence and prognostic impact of tumour cell contamination in autografts. It has been discussed that these contaminating cancer cells could proliferate and induce systemic relapse after stem cell rescue [25]. Even after high-dose therapy with autologous stem cell support, the incidence of relapses with distant metastasis remains a problem. High-risk patients with a potential benefit from additional treatment, such as systemic antibody therapy, should be identified. Here, we present data of patients treated with high-dose therapy and peripheral stem cell support on the single-cell level.

Material and methods

uPA-R expression – clinical samples

A total of 150 samples consisting of bone marrow aspirations (n = 60), peripheral stem cell collections mobilized from steady state haemopoiesis with G-CSF (n = 41), peripheral blood samples (n = 48), and one ascites puncture were obtained from 73 women with breast cancer. A median of one (1–10) sample from each patient was investigated. Thirty-eight samples were obtained from patients with chemotherapy-sensitive metastatic breast cancer, 78 samples from women with primary node-positive disease, and 11 samples from patients with inflammatory breast cancer [15]. For 21 samples stage of disease was not reported.

Additionally, 22 samples from patients without epithelial cancer were investigated. These control samples were bone marrow aspirations (n = 11), leukapheresis samples (n = 8), and peripheral blood collections (n = 3). The donors of these controls suffered from acute or chronic leukaemia (n = 9), lymphoma (n = 11). Eight samples were from healthy volunteers.

Breast cancer specimens and control samples were donated after written informed consent. The protocols were approved by the ethics committee of the Hamburg administration. Mononuclear cells (MNCs) were extracted and counted as previously reported, and subjected to cytospin preparation or immunomagnetic cell selection.

uPA-R expression – immunomagnetic pre-enrichment and immunocytochemistry

The mononucleated cell fraction of the 150 clinical samples was subjected to immunocytochemical stain of cytokeratins without (n = 145) or after (n = 74) immunomagnetic enrichment of epithelial cells with antibodies against the human epithelial antigen (HEA-125) (HEA-Beads, Miltenyi-Biotec, Bergisch Gladbach, Germany) [22]. Immunomagnetic cell selection, preparation of cytospin slides and immunocytochemistry with antibody KL1 or direct-conjugated Fab-fragment A45/B-B3 were carried out as described previously [18,20]. Results from immunocytochemistry prior to and after HEA-selection were combined. The median cell count examined was 5×10^6 with a range from 1×10^5 to $4,02 \times 10^8$. Breast cancer cell lines MCF-7 and MDA-MB453 were used as positive controls and mononuclear cells (MNCs) from non-cancer patients as negative controls. Slides were evaluated by light-microscopy, and positive cells were counted.

The urokinase-like plasminogen activator receptor (uPA-R) has been shown to play a role in the invasive process associated with metastasis [2,21]. Therefore, its expression on disseminated cancer cells was chosen as a second marker to demonstrate that HEA-bead selection is an excellent precondition for immuno-phenotyping of micrometastatic tumour cells. Slides from all samples were available for this investigation. Cytokeratin-positive cells were stained with A45-B/B3, as described above. uPA-receptor detection was performed with anti-CD87 antibody, followed by an immunogold reaction [12]. Large-bowel-cancer cell line HT29 was used here as positive control. Cytokeratin-positive cells stained red and a positive immunogold reaction led to a dark/black stain [12].

Tumour cell quantification prior to and after high-dose therapy

A total of 194 specimens consisting of bone marrow aspirations (n = 87), peripheral blood samples (n = 52) and peripheral stem cell collections (n = 55) were obtained from 52 women with nodal-positive breast cancer, 12 women with inflammatory disease and 11 women with chemosensitive metastatic disease, subjected to high-dose therapy with autologous stem cell support. One woman with metastatic disease was subjected to tandem therapy. All women were treated with two to three cycles of conventional chemotherapy prior to stem cell mobilization from steady-state haemopoiesis using G-CSF (6–12 µg/kg/day) over a period of five days. One or two further cycles were given between apheresis and high-dose therapy [30]. Bone marrow and blood samples were obtained prior to stem cell mobilization and between day +30 and +100 after high-dose therapy. Stem cells were usually harvested on two consecutive days; three harvests were rarely necessary. Blood was usually drawn on the day of marrow puncture. Each sample was investigated separately. However, data from consecutive aphereses and from repeated marrow or vein punctures were pooled for the final analysis, where appropriate [18].

Mononuclear cells (MNCs) were extracted either by ficoll-hypaque (Seromed, Berlin, Germany) density centrifugation or by ammonium-chloride mediated red cell lysis. Samples were assigned randomly to ficoll-centrifugation or red cell lysis. Washed cells were counted with a Coulter counter (Coulter-Immunotech, Krefeld, Germany) and subjected to immunocytochemistry. Cytospin slides from each sample were prepared directly after nucleated cell selection. Sample size permitting, additional slides were prepared after immunomagnetic cell selection from nucleated fraction, using an anti-HEA-125 (human epithelial-antigen) magnetic micro bead conjugate for labelling and separation of epithelial cells (Miltenyi-Biotec, Bergisch Gladbach, Germany) [16]. Cytokeratin-positive cells were detected with antibody KL1 (Coulter-Immunotech, Krefeld, Germany) or with Fab-fragment A45-B/B3 conjugated to alkaline phosphatase (Mikromet, Munich, Germany). Labelled cells were detected either using a biotinylated secondary antibody (primary antibody KL1) and a streptavidine-alkaline-phosphatase complex mediated colour reaction or by using an Fab-fragment directly conjugated to alkaline phosphatase (A45-B/B3) and subsequent colour reaction. Breast cancer cell lines MCF-7 and MDA-MB453 were used as positive controls and mononuclear cells (MNCs) from non-cancer patients as negative controls. Slides were evaluated by light microscopy; the positive cells were counted. A nominal positive result was defined by detection of at least one CK-positive cell [16]. To allow a comparison of quantitative data, the tumour cell load (TCL) per million nucleated cells was calculated for each sample according to the following formula: TCL = (absolute tumour cell count) / $NC_{investigated}$ x10^6 (NC = nucleated cells). Cytokeratin-19 reverse transcriptase polymerase chain reaction was carried out as described previously [17]. Samples investigated by immuno-cytochemistry and rtPCR were found positive when at least one test showed a positive reaction. Samples from volunteer healthy donors served as negative controls, both in immunocytochemistry and rtPCR assays. All samples were obtained after written informed consent. Data were collected using the computer software MS Office (Microsoft, Munich, Germany) and analysed with WinStat (Kalmia Co. Inc., Cambridge, MA, USA).

Survival analysis

The Kaplan-Meyer survival analysis was performed on a total of 165 samples obtained from 71 women with nodal-positive (n = 56) and inflammatory disease (n = 14). The samples consisted of 72 bone marrow aspirates, 45 peripheral blood samples, and 48 leukapheresis samples. Tumour cell identification was done in 127 cases by immunocytochemistry and in 75 cases by cytokeratin-19 rtPCR, indicating that 37 samples were subjected to both tests.

Results

uPA-R expression

A total of 34% of all samples investigated scored positive for tumour cell detection in single-antibody immunocytochemistry. Tumour cells were detected in 43.3% of marrow samples, 29.3% of leukapheresis samples, and 25.0% of peripheral blood specimens.

The mean tumour cell load in all 51 positive samples was 0.82 (± 1.04) in bone marrow, 0.47 (± 0.49) in leukapheresis, and 0.76 (± 0.82) in peripheral blood. The malignant ascites had a tumour cell content of 10%. There was no statistically significant difference in tumour cell load between specimens of different origin, nor between different stages of the disease as calculated by univariate analysis (least significant difference, LSD).

At least one slide from each sample was available for combined anti-cytokeratin/anti-uPA-R double-stain technique. Using this technique, a median count of 2 (1–142) cytokeratin-positive cells was detected on slides from 15 bone marrow aspirations, 9 leukapheresis samples, 10 peripheral blood samples, and the ascites puncture (n = 35).

For a positive result in the nominal analysis of uPA-receptor expression, at least one cytokeratin-positive cell of each sample had to be stained by anti-uPA-R immunogold technique. uPA-R expression was detected in CK-positive cells from 21 specimens, out of which 35 were scoring positive for cytokeratin. uPA-R-expressing cells were detected among cytokeratin-positive cells in 66.7% of

Table 5.2-1 Nominal detection of uPA-R-expression by cytokeratin-positive cells in double-stained slides. For a positive result at least one CK+ cell of each sample had to express the uPA receptor.

Specimen	n	uPA-R positive	
		(n)	(%)
BM	15	10	66.7
LP	9	3	33.3
PB	10	7	70.0
AS	1	1	
Total	35	21	60.0

BM = bone marrow; LP = leukapheresis samples; PB = peripheral blood; AS = ascites.

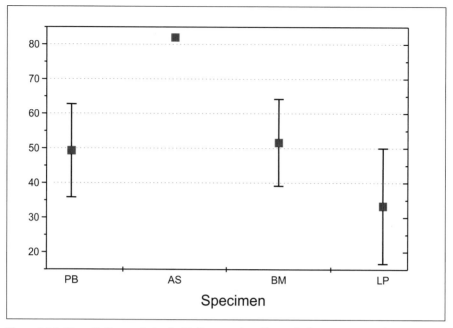

Figure 5.2-1 Quantitative analysis of uPA-R expression. Shown is the percentage of uPA-R-positive cells among cells positive for cytokeratin on double-stained slides (y-axis, mean and standard error bars).
X-axis = samples; BM = bone marrow; LP = leukapheresis samples; PB = peripheral blood; AS = ascites.

bone marrow aspirations, 70.0% of blood samples, 33.3% of leukapheresis samples, and among cytokeratin-positive cells from the malignant ascites (Table 5.2-1). The uPA-R expression was monitored with a significantly reduced frequency in leukapheresis samples as compared to bone marrow (p = 0.03, chi-square), peripheral blood samples (p = 0.02, chi-square), or to all other samples together (p = 0.02, chi-square).

Subsequently, the percentage of uPA-R positive cells among cytokeratin-positive cells was determined. Here, 51.7% (± 48.7) of the tumour cells in bone marrow, 49.3% (± 42.6) of the circulating cancer cells and 33.3% (± 50.0) of the tumour cells detected in leukapheresis samples scored positive. 82% of epithelial cells from the ascites sample reacted with the anti-uPA-R antibody (Fig. 5.2-1). Although the graphic presentation suggests a difference between leukapheresis samples and other specimens, even in this quantitative analysis, the actuarial analysis of the difference does not reach statistical significance (p = 0.15, Mann-Whitney u-test). Neither nominal nor quantitative differences between samples from breast cancer of different stages could so far be detected by univariate analysis (LSD).

Cytokeratin-positive cells could be detected neither by single-stain method nor by combined APAAP/immunogold technique in control samples from patients without epithelial cancer.

Table 5.2-2 Nominal results obtained by immunocytochemistry and cytokeratin-19 rtPCR.

Specimen	BM	PB	LP
pre-HDT (n)	58	34	55
pre-HDT (n+)	31	14	27
pre-HDT (%+)	53.4	41.2	49.1
post-HDT (n)	29	18	
post-HDT (n+)	14	7	
post-HDT (%+)	48.3	38.9	
p (chi-square)	n.s.	n.s.	

Tumour cells prior to and after HDT – nominal results

The nominal analysis revealed a slight decrease of tumour cell contamination after high-dose therapy as compared to the base line from 53.4% to 48.3% in bone marrow and from 41.2% to 38.9% in peripheral blood samples without significant differences (Table 5.2-2). The higher rate of tumour cell contamination in marrow as compared to blood was observed prior to and after high-dose therapy, although without statistical significance (p_{pre} = 0.15, p_{post} = 0.43, chi-square). Tumour cells were detected in 49.1% of autografts. Therefore, the disseminated cancer cells present in the collected bone marrow aspirations would be related to the contamination state of the corresponding stem cell graft. Surprisingly, a tumour-cell negative leukapheresis product predicted significantly the presence of cancer cells in bone marrow after high-dose therapy (p = 0.006, chi-square), (cc: 0.52, p = 0.03, Pearson correlation). Leukapheresis state had no significant influence on nominal detection of circulating tumour cells in blood after high-dose therapy.

Tumour cells prior to and after HDT – a quantitative analysis

High-dose therapy led to a significant reduction in the tumour-cell load of bone marrow from 1.22 (± 1.60) to 0.52 (± 1.32) (p < 0.05, Wilcoxon test). The comparison of tumour cell load in marrow prior to and after high-dose therapy is shown in Figure 5.2-2. TCL decreased after high-dose therapy in all patients, except for one, who showed only a slight increase. In peripheral blood samples, a non-significant increase in tumour cells was observed after high-dose therapy (Fig. 5.2-2, Table 5.2-3). Comparison of TCL values of peripheral blood samples prior to and after high-dose therapy showed equivocal results. Here the kinetics varied (Fig. 5.2-2).

The tumour cell load in marrow aspirations obtained after high-dose therapy was significantly higher in patients without tumour-cell contamination in their stem cell graft (1.07 ± 1.31 *vs.* 0.08 ± 0.17, p = 0.03, Mann-Whitney u-test). However, a high tumour cell load of stem cell grafts did not reciprocally correlate with a high tumour cell load of bone marrow after high-dose therapy (cc = –0.31, p = 0.2, Spearman rank correlation) (Fig. 5.2-3). The same observation was made when the density of circulating tumour cells in the bloodstream was analysed after high-dose therapy. Here again, the TCL was higher after reinfusion of a tumour-cell-free autograft (0.45 ± 0.62 *vs.* 0.002 ± 0.005) but so

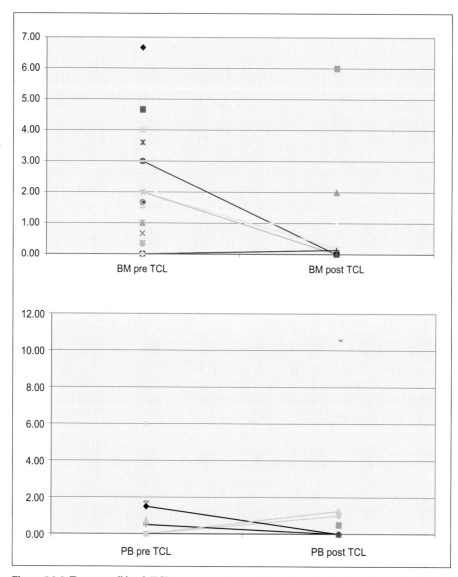

Figure 5.2-2 Tumour cell load (TCL), tumour cells per 106 nucleated cells investigated) in bone marrow (top) and blood (bottom) prior to (pre) and after (post) high-dose therapy with peripheral stem cell support. All data points are plotted, identical points overlap. Pairs from identical patients are connected with lines.

Bone marrow pre TCL = Tumour cells detected per 10^6 bone marrow cells sampled prior to high-dose therapy;

Bone marrow post TCL = Tumour cells detected per 10^6 bone marrow cells sampled after high-dose therapy;

LP TCL = Tumour cells detected per 10^6 leukapheresis cells;

Peripheral blood pre TCL = Tumour cells detected per 10^6 peripheral blood cells sampled prior to high-dose therapy;

Peripheral blood post TCL = Tumour cells detected per 10^6 peripheral blood cells sampled after high-dose therapy;

TCL = Tumour cell load, tumour cells detected per 10^6 investigated nucleated cells.

Table 5.2-3 Tumour cell load (mean and SD) prior to and after high-dose therapy (HDT).

Specimen	TCL pre HDT	TCL post HDT	P
Bone marrow	1.22 ± 1.60	0.52 ± 1.32	P < 0.05
Peripheral blood	0.49 ± 1.22	0.89 ± 2.70	n. s.
Leukapheresis	0.88 ± 1.41	n. a.	

far without statistical significance (p = 0.15, Mann-Whitney u-test). Even here, no correlation was seen between TCL of leukapheresis and blood samples (cc = –0.27, p = 0.2, Spearman rank correlation) (Fig. 5.2-3).

Disseminated tumour cells and prognosis

The impact of disseminated tumour cells in bone marrow – prior to (n = 45) and after (n = 27) high-dose therapy, in blood – prior to (n = 28) and after (n = 17) high-dose therapy, and in leukapheresis samples (n = 48) was calculated by Kaplan-Meyer analysis for disease-free and overall survival. Data from marrow analysis were combined to determine the impact of marrow contamination at any time. Additionally, the impact of disease type (nodal-positive *vs.* inflammatory disease) was calculated to exclude any bias. There was no correlation between the detection of disseminated tumour cells and prognosis in any analysis. For marrow contamination post HDT, there was a trend towards better disease-free survival for women without tumour cells in their marrow, fading after 48 months. The Kaplan-Meyer plot for tumour cell contamination in leukapheresis samples was surprising, because of an obvious trend towards a better DFS for women patients with tumour cells in the harvest, as compared to women with tumour cell negative apheresis.

Discussion

Tumour cell phenotype

The present investigation demonstrates the expression of the uPA-receptor on disseminated breast cancer cells in blood and bone marrow and on tumour cell contamination of peripheral stem cells, harvested after growth factor mobilization. Tumour cells detected in single samples are not phenotypically homogenous. The percentage of cells expressing uPA-R seems to be lower on tumour cells derived from G-CSF-mobilized stem cells (33.3%) than on cancer cells disseminated in bone marrow (51.7%) or circulating in the peripheral blood stream (49.3%). The degree of uPA-R expression was highest (82%) on tumour cells from a single sample of a malignant, secondary ascites invading the peritoneal cavity. However, these differences did not reach statistical significance.

The nominal (black and white) analyses again revealed comparable results for bone marrow and blood specimens, showing here a statistically significant lower expression of tumour cell contamination from G-CSF-mobilized peripheral stem cells.

These results are not attributable to differences between the presence of tumour cells in various specimens or stages of disease. First, in the above

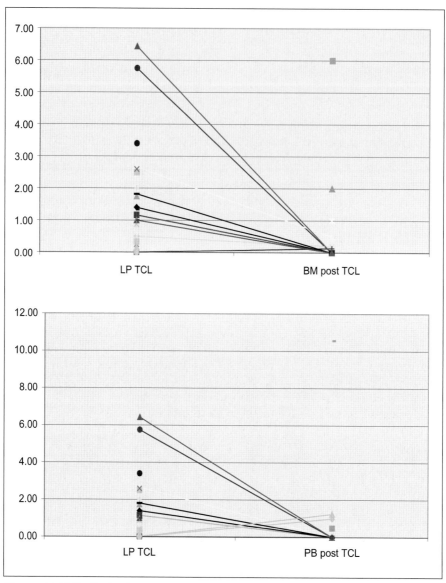

Figure 5.2-3 TCL of leukapheresis samples (LP, left) and marrow (bone marrow, right) (top) or blood samples (peripheral blood, right) (bottom) after high-dose therapy. Samples from identical patients are connected with lines.

Bone marrow pre TCL = Tumour cells detected per 10^6 bone marrow cells sampled prior to high-dose therapy;

Bone marrow post TCL = Tumour cells detected per 10^6 bone marrow cells sampled after high-dose therapy;

LP TCL = Tumour cells detected per 106 leukapheresis cells;

Peripheral blood pre TCL = Tumour cells detected per 10^6 peripheral blood cells sampled prior to high-dose therapy;

Peripheral blood post TCL = Tumour cells detected per 10^6 peripheral blood cells sampled after high-dose therapy;

TCL = Tumour cell load, tumour cells detected per 10^6 investigated nucleated cells.

analysis, only samples positive for cytokeratin in the double-stain technique were included, and, second, preceding large-scale investigation of a median 5×10^6 nucleated cells from each sample excluded significant differences in nominal results and tumour cell load between bone marrow, blood and leukapheresis samples and also between samples from patients at different stages of breast cancer.

Tumour cell mobilization from bone marrow has been discussed, and several attempts were made to kill or remove these malignant cells from autografts by so-called purging procedures [26,27]. This study further shows, for the first time, significant differences in phenotype and pattern of disseminated cancer cells from various provenance. Numerous studies have demonstrated that the plasminogen-activating system plays a central role in the process of invasion and metastasis [13]. Different factors of the system bear a strong relevance for clinical prognosis in breast cancer [14]. The uPA-receptor has been referred to as being essential for migration and invasion of malignant cells [28]. It is not expressed in normal, non-malignant mammary tissue [2]. HEISS *et al.* were able to demonstrate that an increased rate of systemic relapse in gastric cancer patients correlates with the presence of disseminated uPA-R expressing tumour cells, but not to tumour cells lacking the uPA-R [12]. Should circulating breast cancer cells have the capacity to induce or promote systemic relapse, after reinfusion with stem cell graft following completion of high-dose therapy, then the adhesive and invasive capacity of these cells would be a prerequisite for the generation of metastasis. The lower degree of uPA-receptor-positive cancer cells detected in leukapheresis products suggests that the phenotype of these cells differs from the phenotype of disseminated cancer cells found in bone marrow or in normal circulation. Similar uPA-R expression on cells from bone marrow and non-stimulated blood does not support the theory of a down-regulation of uPA-R expression after a mere drift from the bone marrow to the peripheral circulation. One could speculate that disseminated tumour cells found in leukapheresis are less aggressive and have a lower invasive and metastatic capacity than cancer cells present in marrow and non-stimulated blood, owing to a co-mobilization of just less viable or pre-apoptotic cells. Another reason, however, could be a permanent or transient down-regulation of the uPA receptor, as a direct effect of growth-factor administration or as a secondary effect, due to maximal bone marrow stimulation after growth factor administration. As the uPA receptor is not expressed on normal mammary tissue, it can be concluded that malignant breast cancer cells do occur in blood, bone marrow, and leukapheresis products [2]. Furthermore, these results suggest that leukapheresis takes place in a separate compartment for disseminated tumour cell different from marrow and blood. The biological and clinical impact of uPA-R expression on disseminated breast cancer cells will be the object of further research.

Kinetics of tumour cell dissemination

The amount of disseminated breast cancer cells in bone marrow is significantly reduced by high-dose therapy. Complete elimination of tumour cell dissemination in the marrow, however, cannot be achieved in all cases. Surprisingly, the density of circulating tumour cells in peripheral blood shows a non-significant increase after high-dose therapy.

Early tumour cell dissemination in bone marrow has been described in several studies as a negative prognostic factor for disease-free and overall survival. The presence of disseminated cancer cells in the marrow following standard dose chemotherapy is also associated with a significantly higher relapse rate. Most survival curves start to diverge within the first year of follow-up [6,8,11]. The results of the present study do not conform entirely with the data published so far. Neither the marrow state prior to nor after high-dose therapy has any significant impact on survival curves. The trend to better survival of women with, rather then without, tumour-cell positive autografts is surprising. For autotransplantation of metastatic breast cancer, the prognostic impact of tumour-cell contamination could recently be set aside [5]. The authors defined this observation as an effect of the large metastatic tumour burden as compared to the amount of reinfused cancer cells. So far, studies about the impact of disseminated tumour cells, following adjuvant high-dose therapy of non-metastatic breast cancer, are lacking. Mobilization of disseminated tumour cells from bone marrow by different stem cell mobilization protocols has been discussed; and disseminated tumour cells have always been suspected of potentially inducing metastases [4]. The data presented here, and results from two recent publications, would encourage the hypothesis, implying that during growth factor administration used for stem cell mobilization, the co-mobilization of tumour cells will favour less adherent, probably apoptotic tumour cells, to leave the sinusoids of the bone marrow: The presence of tumour cells in the marrow prior to stem cell harvest does not, for certain, predict the contamination of apheresis [19]. The expression of urokinase-like plasminogen activator receptor (uPA-R) , a surrogate marker for a metastatic phenotype, is significantly decreased on tumour cells from G-CSF-mobilized peripheral blood stem cells, as compared to samples of other provenance [29]. So far, the present results clearly show that stem cells as well as bone marrow may harbour different populations of disseminated cancer cells. Furthermore, the clinical data demonstrate that the sole presence of tumour cells in apheresis products is not necessarily associated with a bad prognosis. However, since breast cancer is a tumour known to generate haematogenous metastases, one can at present not completely rule out that tumour contamination of apheresis harbours various cell populations with metastatic capacity. HEISS et al. were able to demonstrate that an increased rate of systemic relapse in gastric cancer patients is correlated to the presence of uPA-R expressing disseminated tumour cells exclusively [12]. Recently, it was, however, shown that disseminated cancer cells are not uniformly either positive or negative as far as the expression of markers with a metastatic phenotype, e.g. the uPA receptor, is concerned [29]. Therefore, future research should focus on the identification of potentially metastatic cell clones amidst the entire population of disseminated cancer cells.

The provenance of micrometastatic cancer cells in bone marrow following high-dose therapy is unclear. There are, principally, at least three theories: (i) Resident dormant , disseminated cancer cells could have survived the high-dose regimen. (ii) Freshly shed cells from the main tumour locations could have repopulated a bone marrow prone to metastases. And (iii), adherence, growing and induction of systemic relapse is induced by tumour cell contamination of stem cell grafts. For haematological malignancies, this has been proven by gene marking studies. In breast cancer, however, analogous experiments have failed so far, owing to the poor transducibility of breast epithelium cells [7,9]. In apheresis, the influence of tumour cell contamination on the detection of disseminated cancer cells after high-dose therapy is surprising. The tumour cell load of bone marrow after high-dose therapy was higher when an obviously tumour-cell free autograft was reinfused. For blood samples obtained after stem cell reinfusion a similar, but non-significant, trend was seen. The marrow data can be discussed as follows: (i) The G-CSF-mediated mobilization of stem cells may have removed disseminated cancer cells from the bone marrow, and tumour cells either have been co-harvested during apheresis or cleared by the immune system. (ii) During apheresis, co-harvested tumour cells may have been immunologically modified by cryoprotectants, freezing and thawing processes. (iii) After their reinfusion, these surface-modified cells induce an immune reaction against other disseminated cancer cells.

In contrast to haematological malignancies, bone marrow is not the home compartment for breast cancer cells. It can therefore be concluded that complete elimination of disseminated cancer cells by high-dose therapy is difficult to achieve. These results would favour the theory that so-called dormant cancer cells survived the standard and the subsequent high-dose therapy and then seeded in the bone marrow as a result of tumour cell contamination after apheresis. Continuing research will be mandatory in order to challenge the hypotheses [3].

Acknowledgements

We wish to thank the Deutsche Krebshilfe (Grant #804) for supporting the clinical trial.

References

1. ALLGAYER, H., et al.: Urokinase plasminogen activator receptor (uPA-R): one potential characteristic of metastatic phenotypes in minimal residual tumor disease. Cancer Res 1997; 57(7):1394–1399.
2. BIANCHI, E., et al.: The urokinase receptor is expressed in invasive breast cancer but not in normal breast tissue. Cancer Res 1994; 54(4):861–866.
3. BRAUN, S., et al.: Lack of effect of adjuvant chemotherapy on the elimination of single dormant tumor cells in bone marrow of high-risk breast cancer patients. J Clin Oncol 2000 Jan ;18 (1):80 18(1):80.
4. BRUGGER, W., et al.: Mobilization of tumor cells and hematopoietic progenitor cells into peripheral blood of patients with solid tumors [see comments]. Blood 1994; 83(3):636–640.
5. COOPER, B.W., et al.: Occult tumor contamination of hematopoietic stem-cell products does not affect clinical outcome of autologous transplantation in patients with metastatic breast cancer. J Clin Oncol 1998; 16(11):3509–3517.
6. COTE, R.J., et al.: Prediction of early relapse in patients with operable breast cancer by detection of occult bone marrow micrometastases. J Clin Oncol 1991; 9(10):1749–1756.

7. DEISSEROTH, A.B., et al.: Genetic marking shows that Ph+ cells present in autologous transplants of chronic myelogenous leukemia (CML) contribute to relapse after autologous bone marrow in CML. Blood 1994; 83(10):3068–3076.

8. DIEL, I.J., et al.: Micrometastatic breast cancer cells in bone marrow at primary surgery: prognostic value in comparison with nodal status. J Natl Cancer Inst 1996; 88(22):1652–1658.

9. DUNBAR, C.E., et al.: Amendment to clinical research projects. Genetic marking with retroviral vectors to study the feasibility of stem cell gene transfer and the biology of hematopoietic reconstitution after autologous transplantation in multiple myeloma, chronic myelogenous leukemia, or metastatic breast cancer. Hum Gene Ther 1993; 4(2):205–222.

10. FIDLER, I.J.: Cancer metastasis. Br Med Bull 1991; 47(1):157–177.

11. FUNKE , I., and SCHRAUT, W.: Meta-analyses of studies on bone marrow micrometastases: an independent prognostic impact remains to be substantiated. J Clin Oncol 1998; 16(2):557–566.

12. HEISS, M.M., et al.: Individual development and uPA-receptor expression of disseminated tumour cells in bone marrow: a reference to early systemic disease in solid cancer. Nat Med 1995; 1(10):1035–1039.

13. JÄNICKE , F., et al.: Both the cytosols and detergent extracts of breast cancer tissues are suited to evaluate the prognostic impact of the urokinase-type plasminogen activator and its inhibitor, plasminogen activator inhibitor type 1. Cancer Res 1994; 54(10):2527–2530.

14. JÄNICKE, F., et al.: Urokinase (uPA) and its inhibitor PAI-1 are strong and independent prognostic factors in node-negative breast cancer. Breast Cancer Res Treat 1993; 24(3):195–208.

15. KRÖGER, N., et al.: Comparison of progenitor cell collection on day 4 or day 5 after steady-state stimulation with G-CSF alone in breast cancer patients: influence on CD34+ cell yield, subpopulation, and breast cancer cell contamination. J Hematother Stem Cell Res 2000 Feb ; 9(1):111–117.

16. KRÜGER ,W., et al.: Immunomagnetic tumor cell selection-implications for the detection of disseminated cancer cells. Transfusion 2000; 40(12):1489–1493.

17. KRÜGER, W., et al.: Reverse transcriptase/polymerase chain reaction detection of cytokeratin-19 mRNA in bone marrow and blood of breast cancer patients. J Cancer Res Clin Oncol 1996; 122(11):679–686.

18. KRÜGER, W., et al.: Tumour cell detection in G-CSF mobilised stem cell harvests of patients with breast cancer. Med Oncol 1999; 16(1):17–22.

19. KRÜGER, W., et al.: Influence of preharvest tumor cell contamination in bone marrow or blood does not predict resultant tumor cell contamination of granulocyte colony-stimulating factor mobilized stem cells. J Hematother Stem Cell Res 2001; 10(2):303–307

20. KRÜGER, W., et al.: Improvement of breast cancer cell detection by immunomagnetic enrichment. Cytotherapy 1999; 1:135–139.

21. MOHANAM, S., et al.: In vitro inhibition of human glioblastoma cell line invasiveness by antisense uPA receptor. Oncogene 1997; 14(11):1351–1359.

22. MOLDENHAUER, G., et al.: Epithelium-specific surface glycoprotein of Mr 34,000 is a widely distributed human carcinoma marker. Br J Cancer 1987; 56(6):714–721.

23. PANTEL, K., et al.: Differential expression of proliferation-associated molecules in individual micrometastatic carcinoma cells. J Natl Cancer Inst 1993; 85(17):1419–1424.

24. PETERS, W.P., et al.: High-dose chemotherapy and autologous bone marrow support as consolidation after standard-dose adjuvant therapy for high-risk primary breast cancer. J Clin Oncol 1993; 11(6):1132–1143.

25. ROSS, A.A. et al.: Detection and viability of tumor cells in peripheral blood stem cell collections from breast cancer patients using immunocytochemical and clonogenic assay techniques [see comments]. Blood 1993; 82(9):2605–2610.

26. ROSS, A.A., et al.: Comparative analysis of breast cancer contamination in mobilized and nonmobilized hematopoietic grafts. J Hematother 1996; 5(5):549–552.

27. SHPALL, E.J., et al.: New strategies in marrow purging for breast cancer patients receiving high-dose chemotherapy with autologous bone marrow transplantation. Breast Cancer Res Treat 1993; 26 Suppl.:S19–23:S19–S23.

28. STAHL, A., and B.M. MUELLER: Binding of urokinase to its receptor promotes migration and invasion of human melanoma cells in vitro. Cancer Res 1994; 54(11):3066–3071.

29. TÖGEL, F., *et al.*: Urokinase-like Plasminogen Activator Receptor Expression on Disseminated Breast Cancer Cells. J Hematother Stem Cell Res 2001; 10(1):141–145.

30. ZANDER, A.R., *et al.*: High-dose mitoxantrone with thiotepa, cyclophosphamide and autologous stem cell rescue for high-risk stage II and stage III breast cancer. German GABG-4/EH-93-Study. Bone Marrow Transplant 1996; 18 Suppl. 1:S24–S25.

5.3 High-Dose Chemotherapy and Autologous Peripheral Blood Stem Cell Transplantation in Four Patients with Neuroendocrine Tumours of Different Primary Sites

Buxhofer*, V., R. Ruckser, P. Kier, K. H. Habertheuer, G. Tatzreiter, P. Zelenka, S. Dorner, Ch. Sebesta, W. Hinterberger

2nd Dept. of Medicine, Ludwig Boltzmann Institute for Stem Cell Transplantation, Donauspital/ SMZO, Vienna, Austria

* To whom correspondence should be addressed (veronika.buxhofer@smz.magwien.gv.at)

Summary

Introduction

The outcome of patients suffering from neuroendocrine carcinoma (NEC) is similar to the clinical course of small cell lung cancer. Even though the initial response to chemotherapy is usually good, most patients experience relapse.

Patients and methods

4 patients with neuroendocrine carcinomas of different primary sites were treated with high-dose chemotherapy (HDC) and autologous peripheral blood stem cell transplantation (aPBSC) as consolidation therapy. Patient #1 had NEC of the lung, patient #2 suffered from NEC of the pancreas, patient #3 presented with metastatic NEC of unknown origin and patient #4 had metastatic NEC of the prostate. After 4–6 cycles of induction chemotherapy, patients received one cycle of HDC consisting of ifosfamide, etoposide and carboplatin, followed by aPBSC.

Results

Patient #1 and Patient #2 achieved CR, and died of relapse 10 and 16 months after aPBSC, that is 16 and 22 months after diagnosis, respectively. Patient #3 is still in CR, with a survival of 38+ months after aPBSC and 45+ months after diagnosis. Patient #4 obtained PR and died of tumour progression 5 months after aPBSC, and 9 months after diagnosis.

Conclusion

Patients with NEC may qualify for HDC and autotransplantation.

Introduction

The prognosis of patients with neuroendocrine carcinoma is comparable with the course of disease in patients with small cell lung cancer, showing a survival of usually less than 6 months without therapy [4,7,10,12,14].

Most reports indicate a good response to chemotherapy consisting of platin and etoposide [9,10,11,13]. We treated 4 patients with neuroendocrine carcinoma with high-dose chemotherapy and autologous stem cell transplantation.

Patients and methods

Patient #1 presented with large-cell neuroendocrine carcinoma that infiltrated the thoracic column. The tumour was radically resected, including laminectomy and resection of the upper lobe of the left lung (R0 resection, TNM staging: pT4pN0M0).

Patient #2 had a carcinoma of the pancreas, 4 cm in diameter, with infiltration of the duodenum (pT3) and lymph node metastases (pN1b). The patient underwent partial duodenopancreatectomy (R0 resection). Histology showed an anaplastic small cell neuroendocrine carcinoma.

Patient #3 presented with a large bulky tumour of the upper abdomen, 8 cm in diameter and with no clearly demonstrable organ connection. The patient had multiple liver metastases so that curative surgery was impossible. A biopsy of the liver revealed an aplastic neuroendocrine carcinoma.

Patient #4 suffered from carcinoma of the prostate, with metastases in lung and bone. Biopsy of the prostate revealed mainly a small-cell, neuroendocrine carcinoma with some small components of adenocarcinoma (Table 5.3-1).

Patients #1–3 received six cycles of chemotherapy consisting of cisplatin (80mg/m^2) or carboplatin (AUC 6) and etoposide (300 mg/m^2 total dose) for induction therapy. Patient #4 received four cycles of chemotherapy consisting of epirubicin (90 mg/m^2) and taxol (200 mg/m^2).

Leukapheresis

Leukapheresis was performed in patients #1, #2 and #3 after the 6th , 5th and 4th cycle of induction chemotherapy with a slightly increased dose of platin. Patient #4 had apheresis after the first cycle of induction therapy. All patients were stimulated with G-CSF (10 γg/kg/d). Apheresis started median on day 14. We carried out three aphereses in patient 1, two aphereses in patient 2 & 3 and four aphereses in patient 4. The yields of CD 34$^+$ cells are listed in Table 5.3-2.

High-dose chemotherapy and stem cell transplantation

Patients received one cycle of high-dose chemotherapy consisting of – total dose – ifosfamide (10 g/m^2), etoposide (1200 mg/m^2) and carboplatin (1200 mg/m^2) on days –6 to –3 for conditioning. After stem cell transplantation, patients were stimulated with G-CSF (5 γg/kg/day) starting on day 8. The respective amounts of transplanted CD34$^+$ cells are listed in Table 5.3-2.

Table 5.3-1 Patient characteristics.

Pat. / age	N.G. / 36	C. SCH. / 36	E.S. / 48	R. SCH. /47 R.
Site	Lung	Pancreas	ABD. BULKY TU.	Prostate
Stage	pT4pN0pM0	pT3pN1bpM	Liver met.	Bone + lung
Histology	Large-CEL NEC	Anapl. small-cell C.	Poorly diff. small-cell C.	Met. mixed (small-cell + adeno.)
Surgery	R0	R0	No	No
Chemotherapy	PE x 6	PE x 6	PE x 6	EPI/ TAXOL x 4

Table 5.3-2 Amounts of transplanted CD34 cells.

			Leukapheresis		Transplantation	
Pat.	Time	No.	CFU-GM 10⁶/ kg	CD-34 10⁴/ kg	CFU-GM 10⁶/ kg	CD-34 10⁴/kg
#1	cycle 6	3	80.85	3.00	61.88	2.14
#2	cycle 5	2	207.49	10.75	118.40	6.13
#3	cycle 4	2	216.71	8.89	41.61	3.43
#4	cycle 1	4	360.86	31.76	2.69	5.57

Results

Haemopoietic reconstitution

All patients engrafted well. Granulocytes increased above 500 G/l on days 10–13.
   One to 4 platelet transfusions and up to 2 red cell transfusions per patient were administered during pancytopenia.

Complications

Side effects were moderate; grade 3 and 4 (according to the WHO classification) side effects concerned emesis and nausea, as well as diarrhoea, and were observed in one patient each.

Outcome

Patient #1 (lung cancer) obtained complete remission after surgery and induction chemotherapy. He relapsed 5 months after aPBSC with brain metastases, and died 5 months later with a survival of 10 months from aPBSC and 16 months from diagnosis, respectively.
   Patient #2 (pancreas carcinoma) achieved complete remission after surgery and induction chemotherapy too. He relapsed 15 months after aPBSC with generalized metastases and died one month later, with a survival of 16 months from aPBSC, and 22 months from diagnosis, respectively.
   Patient #3 (abdominal bulky tumour of unknown origin and liver metastases) achieved partial remission after induction therapy which was converted to complete remission after high-dose chemotherapy. The patient is still in complete remission and in good health with a survival of 38+ months from aPBSC, and 45+ months from diagnosis.
   Patient #4 (carcinoma of the prostate) obtained partial remission after induction and high-dose chemotherapy. He progressed with liver metastases 3 months after aPBSC, and died 2 months later with a survival of 5 months from aPBSC, and 9 months from diagnosis (Table 5.3-3).

Discussion

Neuroendocrine carcinomas, and especially poorly differentiated neuroendocrine carcinomas, belong to a rare tumour entity, without hitherto clear recommendations for therapeutic strategies. Most patients present in advanced tumour stages and in bad clinical condition [4]. Despite satisfactory responses

Table 5.3-3 Outcome.

Patient	Response induction	Response aPBSC	PFS aPBSC	Survival aPBSC	Survival post diagnosis
#1-LUNG	CR	CR	5	10	16
#2-PANCREAS	CR	CR	15	16	22
#3-ABD. BULK.	PR	CR	38+	38+	45+
#4-PROSTATE	PR	PR	3	5	9

to induction chemotherapy, the prognosis remains generally poor with a 2-year survival of less than 20% [10]. Our initial experience with high-dose chemotherapy and autologous stem cell transplantation obtained in 4 patients demonstrates good tolerability, low toxicity and the feasibility of this approach. Comparable to studies on small cell lung cancer [2,3,5], one patient (patient #3) converted from partial remission to complete remission after high-dose chemotherapy. This remarkable patient has remained in complete remission for more than 3½ years. The advantages of intensive induction therapy (smaller tumour load, selection of chemosensitive tumours, improved performance status) has to be balanced against selection and growing of chemoresistent tumour cells which may ultimately cause relapse. Comparable to other tumour entities, a trend towards early consolidation [1,13] and sequential high-dose chemotherapy [6,8] in small cell lung cancer [1,13] is apparent. This approach remains to be further investigated in patients suffering from neuroendocrine carcinoma.

References

1. BRUGGER, W., et al.: Multimodality treatment including early high-dose chemotherapy with peripheral blood stem cell transplantation in limited disease small-cell lung cancer. Sem Oncol (1998) 42–48.
2. ELIAS, A.D.: Dose intensive therapy in lung cancer. In Armitage JO, Antman KH (eds): High-dose cancer therapy. Williams & Wilkins (1996) 824–846.
3. ELIAS, A.D., et al.: Dose intensive therapy for limited-stage small-cell lung cancer: long-term outcome. J Clin Oncol 17 (1999) 1175.
4. HAINSWORTH, J.D., et al.: Poorly differentiated neuroendocrine carcinoma of unknown primary site. A newly recognised clinicopathological entity. Annuals of Internal medicine 109 (1988) 364–371.
5. HUMBLET, Y., SYMAN, M., et al.: Late intensification chemotherapy with autologous bone marrow transplantation in selected small-cell carcinoma of the lung: a randomised study. J Clin Oncol 12 (1987) 1864–1873.
6. HUMBLET, Y., et al.: High-dose Chemo-radiotherapy cycles for LD small-cell lung cancer patients using G-CSF and blood stem cells. Bone Marrow Transplant 18 (suppl) (1996) 36–39.
7. JOHNSON, L.A., et al.: Carcinoids: the association of histologic growth pattern and survival. Cancer 51 (1983) 882–889.
8. LEYFRAZ, S., et al.: Multiple courses of high-dose ifosfamide, carboplatin and etoposide with peripheral blood progenitor cells and filgrastim for small-cell lung cancer: a feasibility study by the European Group for Blood and Marrow Transplantation. C Clin Oncol 17 (1999) 3531–3539.

9. MITRY, E., *et al.*: Treatment of poorly differentiated neuroendocrine tumours with etoposide and cisplatin. Br J Cancer 81 (1999) 1351–1355.

10. MOERTEL, C.G., *et al.*: Treatment of neuroendocrine carcinomas with combined etoposide and cisplatin. Evidence of major therapeutic activity in the anaplastic variants of these neoplasms. Cancer 86 (1991) 227–232.

11. RINDI, G., *et al.*: Gastric carcinoids and neuroendocrine carcinomas: pathogenesis, pathology and behaviour. World J Surg 20 (1996) 168–172.

12. SEITZ, J., *et al.*: Cancers neuroendocrines anaplasiques avances. Bull Cancer 82 (1995) 433.

13. STAREN, E.D., *et al.*: Neuroendocrine carcinomas of the colon and rectum: a clinicopathologic evaluation. Surgery 104 (1988) 1080–1089.

Part Six
Gene Therapy / Immunotherapy in Stem Cell Transplantation

6.1 Shaping the T-Cell Repertoire in Haematopoietic Stem Cell Transplantation and Immunotherapy of Malignant Disease by T-Cell Receptor Transfer

Voss, R. H., F. Schmitz, J. Kuball, C. Lotz, A. Cellary, C. Huber, and M. Theobald*

Johannes Gutenberg University, Dept. of Haematology & Oncology, Mainz, Germany

* To whom correspondence should be addressed (m.theobald@3-med.klinik.uni-mainz.de)

Summary

Selectively shaping the T-cell repertoire in haematopoietic stem cell transplantation and leukaemia immunotherapy towards specific recognition and elimination of malignant and virus-infected cells represents a new therapeutic concept. This concept takes advantage of selectively tolerating or depleting graft-versus-host disease (GvHD) mediating T-lymphocytes, while preserving or selecting cytotoxic T-cell responses specific for malignant and viral disease. Two specific strategies have been extensively explored in preclinical models for this particular purpose (Figure 6.1-1). One strategy is to equip recipient derived T-lymphocytes with "off the shelf" T-cell receptors (TCRs) specific for leukaemia-associated as well as human cytomegalovirus (hCMV)-specific antigenic epitopes, in order to tackle leukaemic relapse and hCMV infection. This strategy is obviously as attractive in immunotherapy of malignant disease, transferring specificity and affinity of TCRs for broad-spectrum tumour and leukaemia-associated antigens into T-lymphocytes of patients and thus breaking their state of cancer and leukaemia-specific T-cell tolerance. Another strategy is to selectively deplete the donor stem cell graft of GvHD mediating alloreactive T-lymphocytes while preserving the integrity of a leukaemia and virus-reactive T-cell repertoire within the stem cell inoculum. As these strategies have been successfully developed at the preclinical level, the opportunity of transferring them into clinical application represents a possible current challenge and endeavour.

Introduction

Progress in conventional and high-dose chemotherapy followed by autologous or allogeneic haematopoietic stem cell transplantation has improved the overall response rate and survival of patients suffering from acute leukaemia. However, a substantial number of patients at defined molecular risk will ultimately relapse after such treatment. There is increasing clinical and experimental evidence that the immune system, and particularly allogeneic cytotoxic T-lymphocytes (CTLs), are able to respond to transformed cells. However, the effect of graft-versus-leukaemia(GvL)-based allogeneic CTL response to malignant disease is

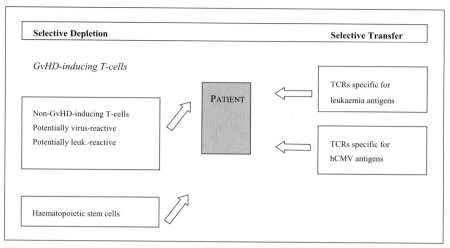

Figure 6.1-1 Shaping the T-cell repertoire in haematopoietic stem cell transplantation and immunotherapy of malignant disease by T-cell receptor transfer.

not specific to neoplastic targets, and is associated with significant toxicity. Obviously, new approaches to treatment are needed.

Adoptively transferring CTLs into cancer-bearing hosts and haematopoietic stem cell graft recipients for the prevention and treatment of malignant and viral disease has been extensively explored in preclinical models and occasionally in man. Although the transfer of melanoma and hCMV-reactive CTLs into patients has been proven therapeutically effective, the widespread clinical routine application of this approach has been jeopardized by logistic and regulatory limitations, not to mention the extraordinary costs of such an entirely individualized cellular therapy [6,12]. As opposed to inducing and generating CTLs with the desired antigen specificities *ex vivo* for each individual patient, the transfer by viral vector transduction of well-defined and "off the shelf" TCR gene constructs with high affinity for broad-spectrum leukaemia and cancer associated antigens and hCMV into T-lymphocytes of stem cell transplant and non-transplant patients suffering from malignant disease represents a promising and more feasible tool for both "state of the art" and large-scale clinical application.

Conceptual Considerations

CTL clones with defined MHC class I restriction pattern, TCR specificity, and functional avidity are an essential prerequisite for any TCR-based transfer strategy. As opposed to hCMV-specific CTLs that can be isolated from patients with viral infection, CTL clones of human origin and specific for defined broad-spectrum leukaemia and cancer-associated epitopes have only rarely been established [1–5,10,11]. HLA-A*0201 (A2.1) transgenic (Tg) mice models have therefore been developed in order to bypass a variety of limiting obstacles, such as mechanisms of self-tolerance as well as low avidity and long-term growth and maintenance of antigen-specific human CTLs generated primarily *in vitro*.

Peptides presented by class I MHC molecules and derived from normal self-proteins that are either constitutively expressed by defined cell lineages or displayed at elevated levels by cells from a variety of human malignancies provide potential target antigens for a universal, CTL-based immunotherapy of haematologic malignancies and cancer. However, as broad-spectrum leukaemia and tumour associated self-proteins are often also expressed at low level in some types of normal tissues, such as thymus, spleen, and lympho-haematopoietic cells, these self-class I MHC/self-peptide complexes are also likely to represent thymic and/or peripheral tolerogens, thereby preventing immune responses. This is particularly true for class I MHC-peptide complexes expressed by bone marrow-derived cells in the thymus, as such expression would cause negative selection of immature thymic T-cells with high avidity for self-class I MHC/self-peptide complexes. The intrathymic deletion of potentially self-reactive T-cells could result in a peripheral T-cell repertoire purged of CTL precursors with sufficiently high avidity to recognize natural leukaemia and tumour-associated self-epitopes presented by class I MHC molecules on malignant cells. Different lines of A2.1 and human CD8 Tg mice provide the basis of an experimental strategy that exploits species differences between human and murine protein sequences in order to circumvent self-tolerance and obtain high avidity A2.1-restricted CTLs specific for broad-spectrum epitopes derived from human self-proteins associated with cancer (p53, hdm2), leukaemia (hdm2), and B cell malignancies (CD19) [7–9].

Preclinical results and discussion

Several antigenic peptides that are naturally processed and presented by A2.1 and correspond to human wild-type (wt) p53, hdm2, and CD19 sequences have been identified in the laboratory. Tg mice-derived CTL lines specific for the identified wt p53 and hdm2 peptide epitopes were of sufficiently high avidity to specifically kill a broad range of A2.1-positive human tumour, leukaemia, and myeloma targets provided that these cells displayed high-level p53 and hdm2 protein expression. In contrast, a variety of non-transformed human cells, such as peripheral blood mononuclear cells, resting T- and B-cells, antigen-activated T-lymphocytes, dendritic cells, fibroblasts, and epithelial cells, all of them which did not express detectable amounts of p53 and hdm2 proteins, were not susceptible to lysis by these CTLs. Similar observations have been made for A2.1-restricted and CD19 peptide-specific CTLs. The anticipation that the self-A2.1-restricted human T-cell repertoire is in fact devoid of such broad-spectrum and high-avidity leukaemia and tumour-reactive CTLs has been confirmed in the laboratory by taking further advantage of a variety of experimental model systems including p53$^{(-/-)}$ mice interbred with A2.1-transgenics [8].

In situations in which the host immune system is devoid of such high-avidity tumour and leukaemia-reactive CTLs, the murine genes for A2.1-restricted and p53, hdm2, or CD19 epitope-specific TCRs could be transferred into patient T-cells. Full length high-affinity αβ TCRs obtained from tumour and leukaemia-reactive Tg CTLs specific for A2.1-presented p53 and hdm2-derived epitopes have been cloned (p53, hdm2) and molecularly modified (hdm2) in the laboratory in order to transfer antigen specificity. Constant regions of human origin have been employed to partially humanize hdm2 peptide-specific TCRs, thereby allowing the prevention or impairment of potential immune responses directed against human T-lymphocytes that express Tg mice-derived double-chain TCR molecules during putative therapeutic intervention *in vivo*.

Each of the hdm2-specific murine wt and chimeric TCR α and β gene constructs was cloned into the pBullet retroviral vector and delivered along with vectors encoding for *gag-pol* (pHIT60) and *env* (pCOLT-GALV) into the 293T packaging line. Human peripheral blood lymphocytes were activated and transduced with wt and chimeric αβ TCRs upon coculture with transfected 293T-cells. Staining of activated human T-cells with a monoclonal antibody (mAb) recognizing the murine Vβ subfamily domains of hdm2, and p53-specific TCRs revealed transduction efficiencies of about 10% to 30%. The non-selected bulk of TCR transduced human CTLs was able to specifically kill peptide-pulsed T2 targets as well as hdm2 and p53-transfectants, albeit less efficiently. The peptide-specific lytic activity of human T-cells derived from different donors and transduced with wt murine and humanized chimeric double-chain TCRs was inhibited in a dose-dependent and specific fashion by anti-murine Vβ subfamily-reactive mAbs. Consistent with this finding, transduction of human T-lymphocytes with either mock or TCR single-chains did not result in antigen-specific CTL responses. This indicated that only the pairing of transduced TCR αβ chains was able to transfer antigen specificity into recipient T-cells. Bulk CTLs were enriched for the relevant murine Vβ subfamily-positive T-lymphocytes in order to increase the quantity of antigen-specific effector cells. These TCR-transduced human CTLs were highly effective in their specific and selective killing of a wide variety of A2.1-positive malignant target cells (Figure 6.1-2 and data not shown). Consistent with the recognition of naturally presented A2.1/peptide complexes on leukaemia and cancer targets was the

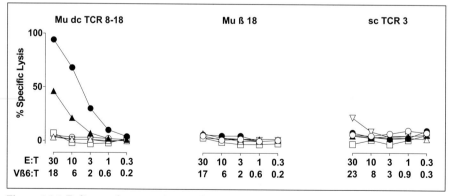

Figure 6.1-2 Delivery of transgenic mice derived T-cell receptors into human T-lymphocytes. Human T-cells, transduced with hdm2 81-88 epitope-specific and CD8 x A2K^b Tg mice derived double-chain (Mu dc TCR 8-18) and non-functional single-chain TCRs (Mu β 18 and sc TCR 3), were tested for cytolytic activity in response to non-peptide (○) or peptide-pulsed (●) T2, hdm2- negative Saos-2 (△), Saos-2/cl5 hdm2-transfectant (▲), A2-negative UocB1 (□), and K562 (▽).

observation that double-chain TCR transduced human CTLs were at least as efficient as parental Tg mice-derived effector cells in their response to limited amounts of exogenous antigen pulsed onto T2-cells.

In conclusion, these results demonstrate that affinity and specificity of A2.1-restricted TCRs, selected in Tg mice by circumventing self-tolerance to universal hdm2 and wt p53 derived CTL epitopes, can be successfully delivered into human T-lymphocytes. This, however, is precisely the molecular requirement to rescue the human T-cell repertoire with high-affinity leukaemia and tumour-reactive TCRs that have been lost due to the establishment of antigen-specific self-tolerance.

Patients undergoing allogeneic haematopoietic stem cell transplantation are at risk for reactivating hCMV, which is usually associated with profound morbidity and mortality resulting from hCMV mediated disease, including life-threatening pneumonitis. A high frequency of hCMV reactivation has also been observed in hCMV seropositive patients enrolled in a clinical trial of autologous CD34 positively selected peripheral stem cell transplantation in combination with rituximab mAb for advanced stage B-cell Non-Hodgkin's lymphoma. Although the incidence of hCMV disease is certainly affected by prophylactic and pre-emptive treatment of patients at risk with ganciclovir, antiviral therapy is also accompanied by substantial side effects and all too often jeopardized by late onset of hCMV disease after discontinuation of ganciclovir while other patients at risk never develop disease or reactivate hCMV before sensitive laboratory screening tests become positive. Class I MHC-restricted CTLs specific for endogenously processed and hCMV derived natural peptide epitopes are particularly effective in limiting viral reactivation and disease [6,12]. The hCMV internal matrix protein pp65 has been reported to provide immunodominant peptide antigens for recognition by hCMV-reactive CTLs. As compared to adoptive transfer strategies with hCMV-specific CTLs, the delivery by retroviral vector transduction of gene constructs encoding high-affinity hCMV pp65-specific TCRs into haematopoietic stem cell transplant patients at risk provides an attractive and innovative treatment option.

Acknowledgements

This work was supported by grants to Matthias Theobald from the Deutsche Forschungsgemeinschaft (DFG) (SFB 432 A3), the "Stiftung Rheinland-Pfalz für Innovation", and the MAIFOR program. We gratefully acknowledge the expert contributions by Edite Antunes Ferreira and Ulrike Liewer.

References

1. GAO, L., et al.: Selective elimination of leukemic CD34+ progenitor cells by cytotoxic T-lymphocytes specific for WT1. Blood 95 (2000) 2198.
2. MINEV, B., et al.: Cytotoxic T-cell immunity against telomerase reverse transcriptase in humans. Proc Natl Acad Sci USA 97 (2000) 4796.
3. MOLLDREM, J.J., et al.: Targeted T-cell therapy for human leukemia: cytotoxic T-lymphocytes specific for a peptide derived from proteinase 3 preferentially lyse human myeloid leukemia cells. Blood 88 (1996) 2450.

4. MOLLDREM, J.J., *et al.*: Evidence that specific T-lymphocytes may participate in the elimination of chronic myelogenous leukemia. Nat Med 6 (2000) 1018.

5. OKA, Y., *et al.*: Human cytotoxic T-lymphocyte responses specific for peptides of the wild-type Wilms tumour gene (WT1) product. Immunogenetics 51 (2000) 99.

6. RIDDELL, S.R., *et al.*: Restoration of viral immunity in immunodeficient humans by the adoptive transfer of T-cell clones. Science 257(1992) 238.

7. THEOBALD, M., *et al.*: Targeting p53 as a general tumour antigen. Proc Natl Acad Sci USA 92 (1995) 11993.

8. THEOBALD, M., *et al.*: Tolerance to p53 by A2.1-restricted cytotoxic T-lymphocytes. J Exp Med 185 (1997) 833.

9. THEOBALD, M., *et al.*: The sequence alteration associated with a mutational hotspot in p53 protects cells from lysis by cytotoxic T-lymphocytes specific for a flanking peptide epitope. J Exp Med 188 (1998) 1017.

10. TROJAN, A., *et al.*: Immunoglobulin framework-derived peptides function as cytotoxic T-cell epitopes commonly expressed in B-cell malignancies. Nat Med 6 (2000) 667.

11. VONDEERHEIDE, R.H., *et al.*: The telomerase catalytic subunit is a widely expressed tumour-associated antigen recognized by cytotoxic T-lymphocytes. Immunity 10 (1999) 673.

12. WALTER, E.A., *et al.*: Reconstitution of cellular immunity against cytomegalovirus in recipients of allogeneic bone marrow by transfer of T-cell clones from the donor. N Engl J Med 333 (1995) 1038.

6.2 Selection of Gene-Modified Haematopoietic Cells

Li[1], Z., B. Schiedlmeier[1], S. Peinert[1], A. Carpinteiro[1], O. Frank[1], A. Wahlers[1], S. Hegewisch-Becker[2], J. Düllmann[3], B. Fehse[2], and C. Baum[1,4*]

[1] Dept. of Cell & Virus Genetics, Heinrich Pette Institute, Hamburg, Germany, [2] Bone Marrow Transplantation and Dept. of Oncology & Haematology, Hamburg-Eppendorf University Hospital, Hamburg, Germany, [3] Neuroanatomy, Hamburg-Eppendorf University Hospital, Hamburg, Germany, [4] Dept. of Haematology & Oncology, Hanover Medical School, Hanover, Germany

* To whom correspondence should be addressed (baum.christopher@mh-hannover.de)

Summary

Gene transfer into transplantable haematopoietic cells offers new perspectives in the treatment of malignant, infectious, and metabolic disorders. Improved techniques for retroviral transduction now allow efficient gene transfer in > 10% of repopulating cells. However, the inability to control the expansion of gene-modified cells *in vivo*, after transplantation, still constitutes a severe limitation. Therefore, it is important to investigate the persistence of transgene expression within individual cell clones after engraftment, and to monitor the functional characteristics of their progeny. We have developed novel retroviral vectors that mediate adequate levels of transgene expression in haematopoietic cells. Using these vectors as tools, we went on to develop and evaluate different selection strategies for gene-modified cells. Stem cell experiments in mice suggest that durable multilineage transgene expression can be achieved with a single selection step, which is, however, accompanied by a reduction in the stem cell repertoire.

Introduction

Gene transfer into haematopoietic stem cells offers promising perspectives in the treatment of malignant, infectious, or metabolic disorders. Improved techniques for *ex vivo* culture and retroviral transduction of haematopoietic cells now allow efficient gene transfer in > 10% of repopulating cells. This could be demonstrated using retroviral vectors and subsequent transplantation of gene-modified human peripheral blood stem cells (PBSC) in immunodeficient NOD/SCID mice [14,15], and even in clinical studies [1,17]. When cytokines are limiting during *ex vivo* culture, lentiviral vectors being able to cross intact nuclear membranes show superior gene transfer rates, but their advantage under optimal culture conditions may be marginal [3].

Irrespective of the type of vector used, the inability to control the expansion of gene-modified cells *in vivo*, after transplantation, constitutes a significant problem. The genetically and phenotypically modified population competes with unmodified counterparts originating from the endogenous stem cell pool. When no conditioning is used prior to or after transplantation, the gene-modified graft may thus be diluted more than 100-fold, resulting in an insignificant contribution to long-term haematopoiesis (< 0.1%) [5]. Also, silencing of transgene expression may cause problems. In the mouse, this occurs primarily upon serial transplantation of retrovirally marked cells, and the incidence is dependent on the type of genetic control elements present in the vector [7]. Therefore, it is important to investigate the persistence of transgene expression within individual cell clones after engraftment and to monitor the functional characteristics of their progeny. The ultimate intention is to establish a new type of genetic control over the engraftment and expansion of gene-modified cells *in vivo*, so that the level of chimerism can be adjusted according to the individual requirements of the patient under consideration. Expression of genes mediating cancer drug resistance in stem cells [1,4,13] and the use of phenotypic markers allowing enrichment of transgenic stem cells prior to transplantation [6,9,11,12] are important first steps in this direction.

Materials and methods

Vectors

Retroviral vectors SF1m and SF11tCD34 developed in our laboratory have been described elsewhere [6,8]. SF1m encodes the human multidrug resistance 1 gene (MDR1), SF11tCD34 a natural splice-variant of the human CD34 sialomucin, lacking the intracellular signal transduction domain. Cell culture supernatants containing replication-defective retroviral vectors with a titre between 5×10^5 and 2×10^6 infectious units/ml were prepared following established protocols [16], using either the amphotropic envelope (SF1m) or the glycoprotein of the vesicular stomatitis virus (SF11tCD34).

Mouse experiments

Mononuclear murine bone marrow cells (C57Bl/6) were prepared and transduced *in vitro* to obtain a gene transfer rate of 10–20%, as described [16]. Cells were transplanted via the tail vein at a dose of $1–2 \times 10^6$ per lethally irradiated (10 Gy) recipient. In the experiments using the SF1m vector, donor cells expressed the Ly5.1 common leukocyte antigen (Ly5.1+), while hosts expressed Ly5.2 (Ly5.2+). Here, untransduced Ly5.2+ competitors were added to the Ly5.1+ donor cells prior to transplantation. Peripheral blood was obtained from the tail vein at various time intervals post transplantation. Cells were prepared for flow cytometry using staining protocols that have been described elsewhere [6,16]. MACS immunoaffinity columns were used for enrichment of cells expressing the tCD34 marker, as already described [6]. Animals were kept and experiments were performed according to ethical guidelines in the facility of the Heinrich Pette Institute.

Results

A conditional selective advantage is mediated by the MDR1 vector, SF1m

MDR1 encoded by the SF1m vector mediates resistance to several cytotoxic agents [4,8,10], and therefore may be useful to reduce side effects of cancer

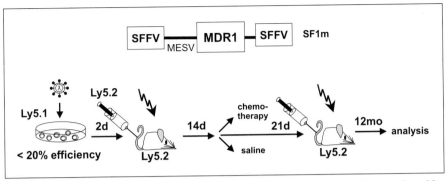

Figure 6.2-1 Experimental strategy to investigate conditional *in vivo* selection mediated by the MDR1 vector, SF1m. SFFV and MESV refer to the regulatory elements of the vector [8,16].

chemotherapy in haematopoietic cells. Mice transplanted with SF1m-modified bone marrow cells and control mice having received a gene marking vector were treated with repeated injections of the antimitotic agent paclitaxel (Fig. 6.2-1). Although only a minor fraction (~ 10%) of repopulating cells contained and expressed the MDR1 transgene (data not shown), the severity of neutropenia induced by paclitaxel was significantly reduced when compared to the controls. The cytotoxicity in the erythroid compartment was also less pronounced. This partial myeloprotection resulted in a clear survival advantage of the SF1m-group (80% vs. 35% in the control group upon treatment with paclitaxel). Notably, serial transplantation of bone marrow cells after chemotherapy produced a shift to donor-type chimerism (Ly5.1+) in bone marrow and spleens of host animals. Presence of the vector SF1m alone, without chemotherapeutic challenge, was not sufficient for this effect. Long-term observation of secondary transplant recipients for up to one year gave no evidence of leukaemic transformation of donor cells (PEINERT, CARPINTEIRO and DÜLLMANN, unpublished data).

Long-term multilineage expression of a cell surface marker, tCD34, from a retroviral vector

The cell-surface marker tCD34, a splice variant of the human CD34 sialomucin, offers interesting features for phenotypic marking and selective enrichment when inserted into blood cells, particularly into T-cells [6]. This marker may also be interesting when targeting primitive CD34– stem cells. To investigate potential side effects that may result from the ectopic expression of this marker in haematopoietic cells, we performed serial transplantations of retrovirally engineered mouse bone marrow cells. The experimental strategy is outlined in Figure 6.2-2. Interestingly, tCD34 allowed multilineage phenotypic marking of transplanted bone marrow cells, equivalent to the widely used cytoplasmic marker, enhanced green fluorescent protein (EGFP). This indicated that ectopic expression of tCD34 did not affect the homing or differentiation of transplanted cells [6]. A follow-up lasting 7 months post gene transfer showed a stable multilineage chimerism in the range of 10% with some interanimal variability. This indicated that tCD34 neither disturbed nor promoted haematopoiesis. For

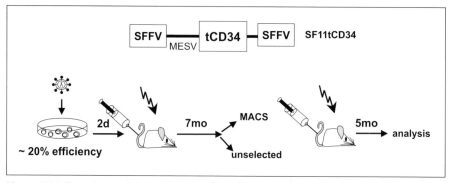

Figure 6.2-2 Experimental strategy to investigate immunoselection and long-term expression of murine haematopoietic cells transduced with tCD34.

serial transplantation, donor bone marrow cells were enriched for expression of tCD34 using immunoaffinity columns or were left untreated. Secondary recipients transplanted with immunoselected cells showed stable multilineage expression of tCD34 in up to 100% of mature myeloid and lymphoid cells, and a similar marking efficiency even in platelets and red blood cells (Fig. 6.2-3). The interanimal variability of tCD34 expression was significantly smaller in the mice which had received immunoselected cells than in those transplanted with unselected ones. This was associated with a small stem cell repertoire in the recipients of immunoselected cells. Some of these mice even presented with monoclonal haematopoiesis, as revealed by Southern blot analysis of retroviral integration sites, and different mice were repopulated by identical stem cell clones, indicating significant expansion of retrovirally marked stem cells in both cohorts.

Discussion

Taken together, the experiments described suggest that transgene expression from improved retroviral vectors such as those developed by our laboratory [4,6,8,16] is (i) maintained over time with a high probability and (ii) of sufficient strength to introduce phenotypic markers operating at the level of trans-plantable stem cells with multilineage potential. Also, the gene-modified stem cells expand significantly in host animals after transplantation, and can be enriched either *in vivo* by drug resistance or *ex vivo* by immunoaffinity, depending on the selection marker encoded. These conclusions are supported by similar findings from other groups, using different selectable marker genes [2,5,9,11 13].

Our experiments were started with a moderate gene transfer efficiency in stem cells (~10 20%). Gene transfer rates in this order of magnitude can be obtained in human PBSC preparations, as documented in NOD/SCID mice and recent clinical trials [1,14,15,17]. Such a moderate gene transfer rate reduces the likelihood of multiple retroviral insertions in single cells, an important requirement for safety reasons. As we have recently demonstrated, higher gene transfer rates may lead to an overestimation of vector performance *in vitro* and

Figure 6.2-3 Example for expression of tCD34 in platelets (Plt) and red blood cells (RBC) 50 weeks after gene transfer, second cohort, recipient of immunoselected cells. Flow cytometry data, blood cells defined by scatter characteristics. The retrovirally expressed human CD34 antigen was detected using a PE-conjugated antibody (BectonDickinson, Heidelberg, Germany).

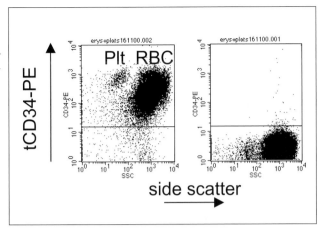

in vivo [16]. Therefore, it is important to note that both markers used here (MDR1 and tCD34) demonstrated the desired properties under the experimental conditions chosen.

Besides revealing encouraging insights into the performance of the vectors and transgenes of interest, the finding of a monoclonal haematopoiesis after a single immunoselection step should also raise a thought of caution. Reduction of the clonal repertoire has previously also been noted after *in vivo* selection by drug resistance [13]. In combination with the strong pressure for forced expansion, this may give rise to complications such as stem cell exhaustion or even transformation to cellular autonomy. However, selection for clonal transgenic haematopoiesis obviously has the striking advantage of allowing faithful multilineage transgene expression with remarkably small variability. Further studies, including carefully designed clinical trials, are required to define the biological limits in this difficult balance.

Acknowledgements

This work was supported by the Deutsche Krebshilfe (10-1456-Ba2, animal models), the BMBF (01KV9811, development of selection systems), and the DAAD (personal grant to Z. L.).

References

1. ABONOUR, R., *et al.*: Efficient retrovirus-mediated transfer of the multidrug resistance-1 gene into autologous human long-term repopulating haematopoietic stem cells. Nat Med 6 (2000) 652.
2. ALLAY, J.A., *et al.*: *In vivo* selection of retrovirally transduced haematopoietic stem cells. Nat Med 4 (1998) 1136.
3. BARRETTE, S., *et al.*: Lentivirus-based vectors transduce mouse haematopoietic stem cells with similar efficiency to moloney murine leukemia virus-based vectors. Blood 96 (2000) 3385.
4. BAUM, C., *et al.*: New perspectives for cancer chemotherapy by genetic protection of haematopoietic cells. In: Expert reviews in molecular medicine (1999).

5. DAVIS, B.M., *et al.*: Limiting numbers of G156A O(6)-methylguanine-DNA methyl-transferase-transduced marrow progenitors repopulate nonmyeloablated mice after drug selection. Blood 95 (2000) 3078.

6. FEHSE, B., *et al.*: CD34 splice-variant: an attractive marker for selection of gene-modified cells. Mol Ther 1 (2000) 448.

7. HALENE, S., *et al.*: Improved expression in haematopoietic and lymphoid cells in mice after transplantation of bone marrow transduced with a modified retroviral vector. Blood 94 (1999) 3349.

8. HILDINGER, M., *et al.*: Bicistronic retroviral vectors for combining myeloprotection with cell surface marking. Gene Ther 6 (1999) 1222.

9. KALBERER, C.P., *et al.*: Preselection of retrovirally transduced bone marrow avoids subsequent stem cell gene silencing and age-dependent extinction of expression of human beta-globin in engrafted mice. Proc Natl Acad Sci USA. 97 (2000) 5022.

10. MICKISCH, G.H., *et al.*: Transgenic mice that express the human multidrug-resistance gene in bone marrow enable a rapid identification of agents that reverse drug resistance. Proc Natl Acad Sci USA. 88 (1991) 547.

11. PAWLIUK, R., *et al.*: Sustained high-level reconstitution of the haematopoietic system by preselected haematopoietic cells expressing a transduced cell-surface antigen. Hum Gene Ther 8 (1997) 1595.

12. PERSONS, D.A., *et al.*: Use of the green fluorescent protein as a marker to identify and track genetically modified haematopoietic cells. Nat Med 4 (1998) 1201.

13. RAGG, S., *et al.*: Direct reversal of DNA damage by mutant methyltransferase protein protects mice against dose-intensified chemotherapy and leads to *in vivo* selection of haematopoietic stem cells. Cancer Res 60 (2000) 5187.

14. SCHIEDLMEIER, B., *et al.*: Quantitative assessment of retroviral gene transfer of the human multidrug resistance-1 gene to human mobilized peripheral blood progenitor cells engrafting in NOD/SCID mice. Blood 95 (2000) 1237.

15. SCHILZ, A., *et al.*: Retroviral-mediated MDR1 gene transfer into NOD/SCID repopulating haematopoietic cells under clinically relevant conditions. Mol Ther 2 (2000) 609.

16. WAHLERS, A., *et al.*: Influence of multiplicity of infection and protein stability on retroviral vector-mediated gene expression in haematopoietic cells. Gene Ther 2001; in press.

17. WILLIAMS D.A., F.O. SMITH. Progress in the use of gene transfer methods to treat genetic blood diseases. Hum Gene Ther 11 (2000) 2059.

6.3 The Chimeric Receptor Strategy. Eliminating Disseminated Tumour Cells: An Immunotherapeutic Approach

Hombach, A., C. Heuser, H. Abken*

Klinik I für Innere Medizin, Labor für Tumorgenetik, Universität zu Köln, Köln, Germany

* To whom correspondence should be addressed (hinrich.abken@medizin.uni-koeln.de)

Summary

A promising approach in adoptive immunotherapy is based on the induction of a specific cellular anti-tumour reaction by antigen-specific, cytolytic T-cells. Due to difficulties in isolating tumour-specific T-cells in sufficient amounts, it was proposed that cytolytic T-cells be grafted with an antigen-specific, recombinant T-cell receptor. The antigen-binding domain of the receptor consists of a single-chain antibody fragment (scFv) that is derived from a monoclonal antibody and binds a tumour-associated antigen. The intracellular signalling domain is derived from the cytoplasmic part of a membrane-bound receptor capable of inducing cellular activation, e.g., the FcεRI receptor γ-chain or the CD3 ζ-chain. By use of this type of recombinant receptor, the strategy combines the advantages of MHC-independent, antibody-based antigen-binding with efficient T-cell activation upon specific binding to the receptor ligand. We designed a panel of recombinant T-cell receptors with specificity for CD30 (Hodgkin's lymphoma, cutaneous T-cell lymphoma), CA19-9, CA72-4, and CEA (adenocarcinoma, gastrointestinal carcinoma), and HMW-MAA (melanoma), respectively. We demonstrated that T-cells engrafted with the recombinant receptor are activated by binding to antigen-positive cells, are not blocked by soluble antigen, and efficiently lyse antigen-positive target cells but not antigen-negative cells. Recent data indicate that induction of IFN-γ secretion and the efficiency of cytolysis by receptor-grafted CTLs is independent of CD28 costimulation, whereas induction of IL-2 secretion by grafted cells requires CD28 stimulation. The chimeric receptor strategy is designed to eliminate disseminated tumour cells by the power of cytolytic T-cells that physiologically penetrate tissues and that are specifically activated by the grafted receptor after binding to antigen-positive tumour cells.

Introduction

The application of immunotherapy to the treatment of tumour metastases has attracted growing interest in recent years. Because of the general belief that T-cell immunity plays a major part in the control of tumour growth, strategies have been recently developed to target and to activate T-cells in a major histocompatibility complex (MHC)-antigen independent fashion towards tumour cells. From the technical standpoint, the strategy can be translated into action by modification of the T-cell receptor (TCR) itself or, alternatively, by

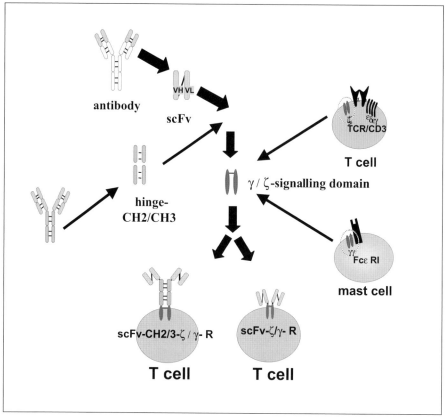

Figure 6.3-1 Generation and expression of recombinant immunoreceptors for use in MHC-independent T-cell targeting of tumour cells.

grafting T-cells with a recombinant receptor. Whereas the first approch requires double transfection of both modified TCR chains into T-cells, ESHHAR *et al.* [3] generated a recombinant receptor consisting of an antibody-derived extracellular domain for antigen-binding and an intracellular signalling domain for cellular activation. By permanent grafting of immunological effector cells with this type of recombinant chimeric T-cell receptor, the strategy bypasses the requirement of presentation of antigen-derived peptides by the major histocompatibility complex to the T-cell receptor complex. Upon antigen-mediated cross-linking, the intracellular signalling domain of the receptor initiates cellular activation resulting in specific cytolysis of the antigen-positive cell (Fig. 6.3-1). The chimeric T-cell receptor strategy combines the effector function of CTLs with the antigen-binding specificity of antibodies. Cellular activation moreover results in limited expansion of receptor-grafted cells that amplify the immune defence towards antigen-positive tumour cells until no cell-bound antigen remains available for sustaining cellular activation. In this situation, the cell is expected to enter apoptosis, thereby limiting the immune reaction.

The chimeric T–cell receptor design

The chimeric T-cell receptor is designed by fusing an extracellular domain for antigen binding with a transmembrane and an intracellular domain for cellular activation. The antigen-binding domain is constituted by a "single chain fragment of variable regions" (scFv) derived from an antibody molecule by joining the V_H and V_L regions via a flexible peptide linker resulting in a continuous polypeptide molecule of the V_H-linker-V_L or V_L-linker-V_H type. The intracellular moiety of the chimeric receptor harbors a signalling domain preferentially derived from the CD3 ζ-chain of the TCR/CD3 complex or, alternatively, derived from the γ-chain of the high affinity IgE Fc receptor (FcεRI) (Fig. 6.3-1).

Taken together, at least three prerequisites enable the design of chimeric T-cell receptors that exhibit both antibody-like specificity and cellular activation capacity:
– an antigen-binding domain with specificity for a membrane-bound antigen;
– antigen-driven, receptor-mediated cellular activation; and
– stable expression of the receptor on the surface of immunological competent effector cells.

During the last years, a panel of chimeric receptors have been constructed with binding domains recognizing human "tumour-associated antigens" (Table 6.3-1). Effector cells transfected with the corresponding chimeric receptor acquire the ability to lyse antigen-positive tumour cells in a MHC-unrestricted fashion (for review see [1]).

The clinical application of the approach needs to comply with at least two prerequisites:
– low immunogenicity of the recombinant receptor molecule to minimize the risk of a host-versus-graft reaction directed to xenogenic parts of the molecule and
– highly efficient transfer of the DNA coding for the recombinant receptor into peripheral blood T-cells and enrichment of the receptor-grafted cells.

Table 6.3-1 Specific T-cell targeting of human tumour cells by chimeric T-cell receptors.

Specificity	Cells targeted	References
ErbB2	breast, ovarian, colon carcinoma	[14,19]
Folate-binding-protein	ovarian carcinoma	[10]
G250	renal carcinoma	[20]
Neu/HER2	breast, ovarian, colon carcinoma	[19]
mIgE	IgE+ lymphoma	[13]
CD30	Hodgkin's lymphoma, cutaneous T-cell lymphoma	[5]
CA72-4	adenocarcinoma	[6,16]
CEA	gastrointestinal carcinoma	[2,8,12,15]
CA19-9	gastrointestinal, pancreas carcinoma	(unpublished)
HMW-MAA	melanoma	[17]
MAGE-A1	melanoma	[22]
CD44v6	metastatic tumours	[4]
KDR	tumour vasculature	[11]
EGP-2	various carcinomas	[18]

The anti-CEA chimeric receptor

The efficacy of the immunotherapeutic approach in targeting tumour cells with effector cells grafted with a recombinant immune receptor is limited by a potential host-versus-graft response against xenogeneic parts of the receptor. To address this issue for use in adoptive immunotherapy of carcinoembryonic antigen-positive (CEA$^+$) tumours, we constructed an entirely humanized T-cell receptor molecule that consists of a humanized, antibody-derived extracellular domain for CEA binding (humBW431/26 scFv), the human IgG1 constant domain as a linker, and the human CD3 ζ-chain for cellular activation [7]. Due to the completely humanized design of the anti-CEA receptor, we do not expect a severe immune response directed against this molecule.

Because retrovirus-mediated gene transfer into peripheral blood T-cells is crucial for efficient expression of the chimeric receptor, we introduced the DNA coding for the humBW431/26-scFv-Fc-ζ receptor into the retroviral vector pSTITCH, which allows highly efficient transduction of T-cells utilizing a transiently packaging system [21]. The retroviral vector was packed into GaLV- and A-MuLV pseudotyped viruses, which utilize different receptors for T-cell entry. After retroviral transduction, we monitored expression of the anti-CEA receptor by FACS analysis utilizing an anti-idiotypic antibody directed to the scFv domain, or, alternatively, an anti-human IgG antibody directed to the extracellular spacer domain of the receptor (Fig. 6.3-2). Monitoring the number of receptor-grafted T-cells revealed that both GaLV- and MuLV-pseudotyped retroviruses efficiently transduce peripheral blood T-cells with nearly similar efficiencies [7]. Given the differences in transduction efficiencies utilizing lymphocytes from various donors, the efficiency of gene transfer more likely

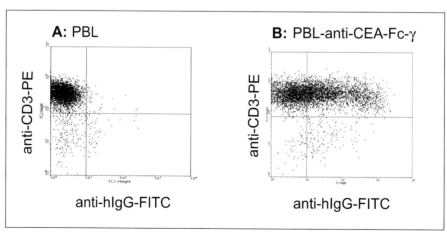

Figure 6.3-2A, B Two-colour immunofluorescence of anti-CEA-γ (BW431/26-scFv-Fc-γ) receptor grafted peripheral blood T-cells.
Non-transduced **(A)** and anti-CEA-γ receptor grafted **(B)** peripheral blood T-cells were simultaneously incubated with a FITC-conjugated anti-human IgG Fc antibody and a PE-conjugated anti-human CD3 antibody, respectively (2 μg/ml each) and analysed by flow cytometry.

depends on the particular blood donor than on the different envelopes used to pack the retroviral vector. This conclusion is of practical relevance, because retroviral transduction of lymphocytes from some donors will consistently result in low numbers of grafted T-cells.

The success of the chimeric receptor strategy likely depends on the absolute number and ratio of receptor-grafted effector cells in a cell population to be administered during adoptive immunotherapy. Low transduction rates due to the individual lymphocyte donor make it necessary to enrich receptor-grafted T-cells before clinical administration. Utilizing antibodies directed against the extracellular constant domain of the receptor, receptor expressing cells can, moreover, be separated by magnetic activated cell sorting (MACS) from non-receptor-grafted cells. By one round of cell sorting, we specifically enriched receptor-grafted T-cells about 2- to 6-fold from a mixed cell population [7]. This procedure is still efficient even when poorly transduced donor lymphocytes are used (< 10% transduced cells). Receptor-grafted T-cells can subsequently be expanded *in vitro* to numbers sufficient for *in vivo* targeting.

Cellular activation

The binding domain of the humBW431/26-scFv-Fc-γ receptor preferentially binds to the membrane-bound form of CEA. Thus, the immune receptor mediates cellular activation preferentially after binding to membrane-bound CEA [8]. Accordingly, T-cells grafted with the anti-CEA-γ chain receptor are activated by membrane-bound CEA even in the presence of high amounts of soluble CEA often found in sera of tumour patients. As an alternative to the γ-signalling chain, we combined the extracellular part of the receptor with the transmembrane and intracellular part of the CD3 ζ-signalling chain that contains three immunoreceptor tyrosine-based activation motifs (ITAM) in contrast to one ITAM of the FcϵRI γ-chain. Like the γ-chain receptor, the BW431/26-scFv-Fc-ζ-chain receptor induces an effective and MHC-independent immune response of grafted T-cells from the peripheral blood against CEA$^+$ tumour cells even at low effector-to-target ratios *in vitro* [7] (Fig. 6.3-3).

CD28 costimulation

According to the two-signal paradigm, resting T-cells can be activated by either crosslinking of the TCR complex in addition to exogeneous IL-2 or stimulation via CD28. The role of CD28 costimulation in activated T-cells is, however, not completely resolved. Once T-cells are activated, the triggering of antigen-specific cytolysis via the TCR/CD3 complex appears to be independent of CD28 costimulation. We most recently explored the role of CD28 costimulation for receptor mediated signalling of T-cells grafted with chimeric receptors [9]. Utilizing a panel of recombinant receptors we found that

- receptor-mediated target-cell lysis is nearly unaffected by CD28/B7-signalling,
- antigen specific IL-2 secretion, but not IFN-γ secretion, requires CD28 costimulation, and
- cellular proliferation of grafted T-cells is increased upon CD28 costimulation.

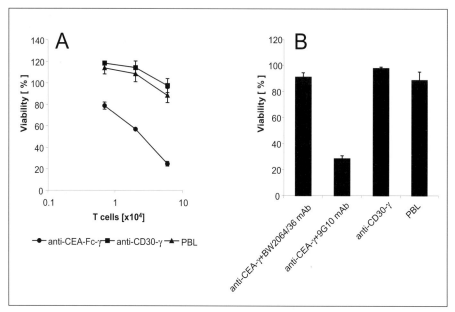

Figure 6.3-3A, B Specific cytolysis of CEA[+] target cells by anti-CEA receptor grafted T-cells.
A: T-cells were grafted with the anti-CEA receptor BW431/26-scFv-Fc-γ and for control with the anti-CD30 receptor HRS3-scFv-γ. Receptor grafted and non-transduced T-cells (0.7 x 10⁴ - 6 x 10⁴ cells/well) were cocultivated for 48 h with CEA[+] Lovo tumour cells (5 x 10⁴ cells/well) in 96-well tissue culture plates.
B: To demonstrate specificity of receptor mediated cell lysis, anti-CEA- and anti-CD30-receptor grafted T-cells were cocultivated with CEA[+] Lovo tumour cells (5 x 10⁴ cells/well) in 96-well tissue culture plates for 48 h in the presence of the anti-CEA receptor specific anti-idiotypic mAb BW2064/36 and an IgG1 control mAb (9G10), respectively (each 10 μg/ml).
Specific cytotoxicity was monitored by a XTT-based colorimetric assay (Roche Diagnostics, Mannheim, Germany) as described by JOST et al., J Immunol Meth 147 (1992) 153–165. The proportions of anti-CEA- and anti-CD30 receptor grafted T-cells were 20.5% and 12.84%, respectively. The assay was done in triplicate. SEM = standard error of means.

This demonstrates that cytokine secretion and proliferation are at least partially uncoupled from the capacity to lyse target cells.

The results have substantial consequences for the concept of MHC-independenT-cellular targeting by recombinant receptor molecules:

– Cytolysis of antigen-positive tumour cells by receptor-grafted T-cells is efficient even when costimulatory molecules are missing on the target cells. This is of importance since most tumour cells do not provide CD28 costimulation.

– IL-2 secretion by receptor-grafted T-cells requires CD28 costimulation. Since IL-2 plays a key role for Th1-based cellular immunity, targeting of tumour cells lacking costimulatory molecules by receptor-grafted T-cells will only result in a limited cellular immune response. On the other hand, IL-2, secreted in high concentrations by grafted, activated T-cells into the tumour microenvironment, may be effective in attracting of a second wave of nonspecific inflammatory cells, thus locally enhancing the anti-tumour effect and eradicating antigen-negative tumour cells. In the absence of CD28 costimulation and despite high IFN-γ secretion levels, the acquisition of additional cellular effectors, e. g. natural killer cells, and the maintenance of a prolonged anti-tumour reactivity of receptor-grafted T-cells requires CD28 costimulation.

– CD28 costimulation modulates cytokine secretion upon crosslinking of the recombinant receptor as well as of the CD3/TCR complex. We conclude that cellular activation of grafted T-cells via the recombinant receptor is regulated and integrated in a similar fashion as T-cell activation via the common CD3/TCR complex.

Taken together, CD28 costimulation obviously co-modulates cell activation parameters independently of each other, i.e., cytokine secretion, proliferation, and cytolysis. Due to a highly variable expression pattern of these molecules on target cells, the requirement of costimulation has substantial consequences for the efficiency of the cellular immune response against target cells using cytotoxic T-cells equipped with either the native or a grafted recombinant T-cell receptor.

Conclusions and perspectives

Recombinant immunoreceptors are designed to constitute a strategy for cellular immunotherapy that bypasses the MHC restriction of antigen recognition. T-cells grafted with the receptor are activated upon antigen-specific receptor crosslinking in a MHC-independent fashion and mediate efficiently a cellular immune response against antigen-positive tumour cells. Entirely humanized receptors are required for clinical applications in order to prevent the efficacy of the approach from being limited by a potential host-versus-graft response against xenogeneic parts of the receptor.

One of the major hurdles of the strategy is the intrinsic heterogeneity of antigen expression within the malignancy. Whereas antigen-positive tumour cells may be successfully eliminated by receptor-grafted, cytolytic T-cells, antigen-negative tumour cells will not be recognized by the grafted receptor. This potential limitation might be overcome by utilizing populations of effector cells transfected with chimeric receptors recognizing different antigens of the same tumour.

A beneficial effector-cell to target-cell ratio at the tumour site is likely to be required for efficient target T-cell lysis. An estimation based on clinical data, however, is not yet available. We assume that systemic application of about 10^8 receptor-grafted cells is likely to be necessary for efficient elimination of residual tumour cells *in vivo*. This situation requires a prolonged lymphocyte expansion *in vitro* prior to application *in vivo*, a high proportion of lymphocytes effectively transduced, and a stable expression of the receptor on the cell surface.

Other types of effector cells, e.g., natural killer cells or macrophages, may be as effective as CTLs or may act synergistically when administered together with receptor-grafted CTLs. Due to the modular composition of the receptor molecule, the antigen-binding domain may be combined for this reason with a particular signalling domain that is required for the particular effector cell.

Immunotherapeutic approaches that rely exclusively on the induction and/or redirection of cytotoxic T-cell responses are frequently of limited value in clinical situations accompanied by immunosuppression. Therefore, problems may arise with the clinical situation of the individual patient.

Taken together, the stable genetic modification of immunocompetent effector cells harbours the potential to extend the current scope of adoptive cellular immunotherapy by combining MHC-independent tumour cell recognition with the cytolytic activity of effector cells. Although questions remain, clinical trials likely to be implemented in the near future will determine the feasibility of the strategy in countering the escape of tumour cells from immune surveillance.

Acknowledgements

Work in the author's laboratories is supported by grants from the Deutsche Forschungsgemeinschaft, the SFB502, the Deutsche Krebshilfe, and the Köln Fortune programme.

References

1. ABKEN, H., *et al.*: Can combined T-cell-antibody-based immunotherapy outsmart tumour cells? Immunology Today 19 (1998) 2–5.
2. DARCY, P.K., *et al.*: Expression in cytotoxic T-lymphocytes of a single-chain anti-carcinoembryonic antigen antibody: redirected Fas ligand-mediated lysis of colon carcinoma. Eur J Immunol 28 (1998) 1663–1672.
3. ESHHAR, Z., *et al.*: Specific activation and targeting of cytotoxic lymphocytes through chimeric single chains consisting of antibody-binding domains and the gamma or zeta subunits of the immoglobulin and T-cell receptors. Proc Natl Acad Sci USA 90 (1993) 720–724.
4. HEKELE, A., *et al.*: Growth retardation of tumours by adoptive transfer of cytotoxic T-lymphocytes reprogrammed by CD44v6-specific scFv:zeta-chimera. Int J Cancer 68 (1996) 232–238.
5. HOMBACH, A., *et al.*: An anti-CD30 chimeric receptor that mediates CD3-ζ independent T-cell activation against Hodgkin's lymphoma cells in the presence of soluble CD30. Cancer Res 58 (1998) 1116–1119.
6. HOMBACH, A., *et al.*: T-cell targeting of TAG72+ tumour cells by a chimeric receptor with antibody-like specificity for a carbohydrate epitope. Gastroenterol 113 (1997) 1163–1170.
7. HOMBACH, A., *et al.*: An entirely humanized CD3 z-chain signalling receptor that directs peripheral blood T-cells to specific lysis of carcinoembryonic antigen-positive tumour cells. Int J Cancer 88 (2000) 115–120.
8. HOMBACH, A., *et al.*: A chimeric receptor that selectively targets membrane-bound carcinoembryonic antigen (mCEA) in presence of soluble CEA. Gene Ther 6 (1999) 300–304.
9. HOMBACH, A., *et al.*: T-cell activation by recombinant receptors: CD28 costimulation is required for IL-2 secretion and receptor mediated T-cell proliferation but does not affect receptor-mediated target-cell lysis. Cancer Res 61 (2001) 1976–1982.
10. HWU, P., et al.: Lysis of ovarian cancer cells by human lymphocytes redirected with a chimeric gene composed of an antibody variable region and the Fc receptor g chain. J Exp Med 178 (1993) 361–366.
11. KERSHAW, M.H., *et al.*: Generation of gene-modified T-cells reactive against the angiogenic kinase insert domain-containing receptor (KDR) found on tumour vasculature. Hum Gene Ther 11 (2000) 2445–2452.
12. KUROKI, M., *et al.*: Specific targeting strategies of cancer gene therapy using a single-chain variable fragment (scFv) with a high affinity for CEA. Anticancer Res 20 (2000) 4067–4071.

13. LUSTGARTEN, J., Z. ESHHAR: Specific elimination of EgE production using T-cell lines expressing chimeric T-cell receptor genes. Eur J Immunol 25 (1995) 2985–2991.

14. MORITZ, D., *et al.*: Cytotoxic T-lymphocytes with a grafted recognition specificity for ErbB2-expressing tumour cells. Proc Natl Acad Sci USA 91 (1994) 4318–4322.

15. NOLAN, K.F., *et al.*: Bypassing immunization: optimized design of "designer T-cells" against carcinoembryonic antigen (CEA)-expressing tumours, and lack of suppression by soluble CEA. Clin Cancer Res 5 (1999) 3928–3941.

16. PATEL, S.D., *et al.*: Anti-tumour CC49-zeta CD4 T-cells possess both cytolytic and helper functions. J Immunother 23 (2000) 661–668.

17. REINHOLD, U., *et al.*: Specific lysis of melanoma cells by receptor-grafted T-cells is enhanced by anti-idiotypic monoclonal antibodies directed to the scFv domain of the receptor. J Invest Dermatol 112 (1999) 101–108.

18. REN-HEIDENREICH, L., *et al.*: Specific targeting of EGP-2+ tumour cells by primary lymphocytes modified with chimeric T-cell receptors. Hum Gene Ther 11 (2000) 9–19.

19. STANCOVSKI, S., *et al.*: Targeting of T-lymphocytes to Neu/Her2-expressing cells using chimeric single chain Fv receptors. J Immunol 151 (1993) 6577–6582.

20. WEIJTENS, M.E., *et al.*: Single chain Ig/gamma gene-redirected human T-lymphocytes produce cytokines, specifically lyse tumour cells, and recycle lytic capacity. J Immunol 157 (1996) 836–843.

21. WEIJTENS, M.E., *et al.*: A retroviral vector system "STITCH" in combination with an optimized single-chain antibody chimeric receptor gene structure allows efficient gene transduction and expression in human T-lymphocytes. Gene Ther 5 (1998) 1195–1203.

22. WILLEMSEN, R.A., *et al.*: Grafting primary human T-lymphocytes with cancer-specific chimeric single-chain and two-chain TCR. Gene Ther 7 (2000) 1369–1377.

6.4 Suicide Gene Therapy for GvHD

Fehse[1]*, B., Z. Li[2], K. Kühlcke[3], L. Fang[1], O. S. Kustikova[1], F. Ayuk[1], A. A. Fauser[4], H.-G. Eckert[3], C. Baum[2,5], A. R. Zander[1]

[1] Bone Marrow Transplantation, Hamburg-Eppendorf University Hospital, Hamburg,
[2] Heinrich Pette Institute for Experimental Virology and Immunology, Hamburg,
[3] EUFETS Idar-Oberstein, [4] Clinics for BMT Idar-Oberstein, [5] Dept. of Haematology and Oncology, Hanover Medical School, Germany

* To whom correspondence should be addressed (fehse@uke.uni-hamburg.de)

Summary

A new concept for the management of graft-versus-host disease (GvHD) recently developed by TIBERGHIEN *et al.* and BORDIGNON *et al.* is based on the introduction of a suicide gene (e.g. Herpes simplex virus thymidine kinase, HSV-tk) into allogeneic donor T-lymphocytes. In case of GvHD onset, activation of the suicide mechanism by administration of the antiviral drug ganciclovir allows selective depletion of alloreactive T-cells. After first *proof of principle-* clinical studies, further development of this strategy is necessary in order to enable its broad clinical application.

Introduction

T-lymphocytes play an important role in allogeneic haematopoietic stem cell transplantation (HSCT) by supporting transplant engraftment and immune recovery of the patient. Most remarkably, donor T-cells exert an immunological reaction against remaining malignant T-cells, an effect now well-known as the *graft-versus-leukaemia* (GvL) reaction. The power of the latter was impressively shown by the pioneering work of KOLB, SLAVIN and their colleagues [17,23] who established the concept of adoptive immunotherapy based on donor leukocyte (or lymphocyte) infusions (DLI). Meanwhile, DLI have become a real treatment option in the context of allogeneic HSCT, to cure not only leukaemic relapses [17,23] but also life-threatening infections [19,21]. However, allogeneic T-lymphocytes may also direct their cytotoxic potential against healthy tissue of the patient, a graft-versus-host reaction (GvHR) that can lead to a severe, potentially lethal disease (GvHD).

Consequently, lots of efforts have been made to separate GvL from GvH reactions – or to, at least, control GvHD. This seems to be possible, because strong antileukaemic reactions have been reported in the absence of acute GvHD [2]. First concepts were based on T-cell depletion (TCD) with delayed add-back of defined T-cell numbers. Later, defined T-cell subsets (e.g. CD4, CD5, CD6, CD8) were depleted using monoclonal antibodies (AB). This has, however, led to controversial results regarding the importance of one or the other cell population for GvL and GvH reactions [for ref.: 8]. Alternatively, *ex vivo* activation of alloreactive T-cells and elimination of CD25- (= IL-2 receptor α-chain) expressing cells using immunotoxins has been suggested [for ref.: 8]. More recently, we and others developed strategies using magnetic cell sorting

Table 6.4-1 Clinical studies on the use of suicide gene-modified T-lymphocytes for controlling GvHD.

	BORDIGNON	CHAMPLIN	TIBERGHIEN
Infusion of gene-modified cells	DLI	DLI	Co-infusion with TCD-BM
Diagnosis	Relapse or EBV lymphoma	Relapse	Haematological malignancy indicating allogeneic BMT
Number of patients	8	23	12
Number of infused T-cells	0.5–40 x 106/kg RW Min. dose for EBV: 1 x 10⁶/kg	0.7–190 x 106/kg RW (1–4 doses)	2, 6 or 20 x 106/kg RW
Clinical outcome	3 CR, 2 PR, 2 NR, 1 NE	2 CR, 4 SD, 17 PD	CML: 3/4 alive in CR AML: 1/2 alive in CR 3 EBV lymphomas
GvHD treatment with ganciclovir alone	Effective in 2 cases of aGvHD, 1 failure in cGvHD	Only 1 GvHD-resolved w/o treatment	Effective in 2/3 cases with aGvHD and in 1 case with cGvHD
Source	[8]	[9]	[10]

CR = complete response, PR = partial response, NR = no response, NE = not evaluable, SD = stable disease, PD = progressive disease, TCD = T-cell depletion, RW = recipient's weight

to deplete cells expressing activation-induced antigens (CD25, CD69) after alloactivation [8]. All these strategies have been subjects of clinical trials (or such trials are in preparation) highlighting the importance of the problem.

A few years ago two groups independently suggested a gene therapy approach to control graft-versus-host disease (GvHD) [4,24]. This strategy is based on the introduction of a "suicide gene" into T-cells allowing their *in vivo* elimination in the event of GvHD. Relying on this concept, at least three clinical studies [4,5,25] have been carried out so far, the results of which are summarized in Table 6.4-1. The following conclusions could be drawn from the results of these studies: (1) Infusion of suicide gene-modified T-cells is feasible and safe, (2) GvL has been obtained without GvHD in some patients, (3) T-cell function seems to be reduced as a result of *ex vivo* culture, (4) T-cell depletion led to a high incidence of EBV-associated lymphoproliferative disease and (5) Current gene transfer techniques (including efficacy of transgenes used so far) have not been to everyone's satisfaction: low gene transfer efficiencies, long *in vitro* culture for selection, impaired suicide mechanism in 2 of 7 patients due to non-functional HSV-tk variants (see below).

In the light of these results, several improvements are necessary to secure further application of adoptive immunotherapy with suicide gene-modified T-cells. In particular, improved retroviral vectors which ensure sufficient and stable expression of both the suicide gene and the positive selection marker are required. Also, more efficient transduction protocols which could be used in accordance with the rules of "good manufacturing practice" (GMP) should be developed. These protocols should enable conservation of maximal T-cell function after *ex vivo* culture. Introduction of alternative selection markers could shorten the time required for *ex vivo* culture. Improved suicide mechanisms should guarantee almost 100% killing of alloreactive T-cell clones. Finally, subsequent clinical studies should be designed after thorough analysis of the clinical experience accumulated in the trials completed so far.

We have devised a multi-centre clinical phase I/II study on the use of gene-modified T-lymphocytes in allogeneic bone marrow/peripheral blood stem cell transplantation which is expected to be initiated in 2001. In preparation for this study we have developed a research programme addressing several of the issues mentioned above.

Results and discussion

Clinical study

A phase I/II multicentre clinical study "The use of gene-modified donor T-cells in allogeneic bone marrow transplantation (BMT) and peripheral blood stem cell transplantation (PBSCT)" (Fig. 6.4-1) has been designed by A. R. ZANDER, B. FEHSE, A. A. FAUSER and W. I. BLAU. During finalization, the study design has also been discussed with our Swedish colleagues S. DILBER and J. ASCHAN who will perform the study at Huddinge University Hospital.

The protocol, like the strategy described by TIBERGHIEN *et al.* [25], proposes gene-modified T-cells to be co-infused with the T-cell-depleted stem cell graft. In contrast to that study, T-cell depletion will be carried out by CD34-enrichment, allowing co-depletion of B-cells. This may be of significance, considering the EBV-lymphoma cases in TIBERGHIEN's study (Table 6.4-1).

A target value of 5×10^6/kg recipient's weight (minimum: 1×10^6/kg) gene-modified T-cells will be infused together with the CD34$^+$ cells. This relatively high cell number takes into account the reports of impaired T-cell function mentioned in relevant studies. To increase the probability of an efficient GvL reaction, an optional second infusion of gene-modified T-cells is scheduled at day 60 post transplantation.

The chief objective of our study is to evaluate safety and toxicity of gene-modified donor T-cells given together with donor CD34-enriched haemato-poietic stem cells from peripheral blood or bone marrow. Further objectives include the evaluation of (i) survival and function of the gene-modified cells in peripheral blood, (ii) their survival after ganciclovir treatment, (iii) thereafter, the incidence, response and severity of graft-versus-host disease, and (iv) engraftment and relapse rates.

The study is expected to start in 2001, both in Germany and in Sweden. In conjunction with the preparation of the study, our laboratories joined forces in order to define the technological prerequisites for a successful implementation.

Retroviral vectors

We developed new retroviral hybrid vectors in our laboratories, in which the U3 region of MESV has been replaced by the stronger promotors of myelo-proliferative sarcoma virus (MPSV) and spleen focus forming virus (SFFV) [3,7]. Thorough mapping of existing and inclusion of alternative control elements,

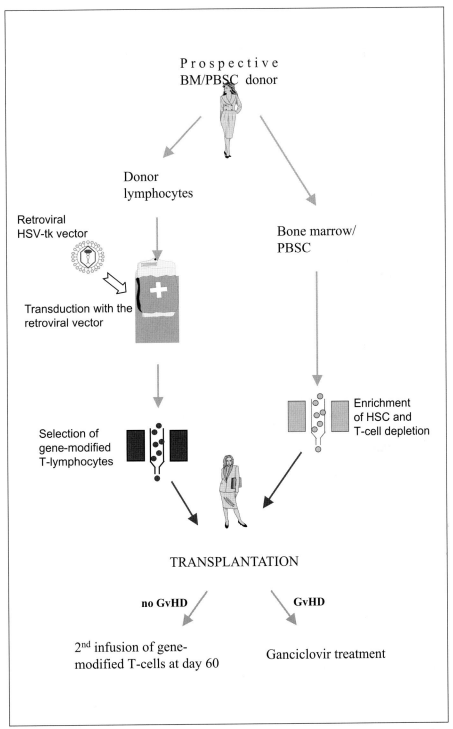

Figure 6.4-1 Clinical study on the use of suicide gene-modified T-cells-outline. In the first study described here, selection of transduced cells will be based on neomycin resistance.

such as the post-transcriptional regulatory element (PRE) from Woodchuck hepatitis virus, now enables the design of vectors predominantly active in T-lymphocytes [reviewed in 3]. We also used different linkage strategies, in order to ensure high expression of two transgenes [14,15]. Recently, new vectors which utilize cotranslational protein separation were developed in our laboratories [16].

Transduction protocols and *ex vivo* culture

The first study with gene therapy, in which suicide gene-modified T-cells were used, exploited co-cultivation to obtain sufficient gene transfer [4]. This method remains controversial, because of safety problems. Therefore, in 1998, we and others presented protocols for highly efficient gene transfer into human primary T-lymphocytes using retroviral supernatant on fibronectin [9,20]. Subsequently, our protocol has further been improved for clinical application. In particular, it avoids the use of foetal bovine serum (FBS) in all cell culture steps during transduction [1]. We have now developed a protocol based on pre-loading cell culture vessels with retroviral vectors. Besides very high transfer efficiencies, this strategy has several additional advantages: It neither requires fibronectin-coating (which may interact with cellular physiology, and is quite expensive) nor centrifugation of target cells during transduction. Moreover, any target cell can be cultured and transduced in its optimal medium [KÜHLCKE *et al.*, submitted; ECKERT *et al.*, see Chapter 6.5, page 204].

Clinical results (see above), as well as *in vitro* and *in vivo* experiments, suggest that T-cell function may be heavily impaired after prolonged *ex vivo* culture [reviewed in AYUK *et al.*, submitted]. Alternative stimulation of primary T-cells with OKT3/CD28 not only ensures optimal proliferation but seems to also prevent alterations in the T-cell repertoire [12]. Indeed, using *in vitro* assays, we found alloreactivity to be conserved to a high extent for at least one week after stimulation with immobilized OKT3/α-CD28 antibodies (not shown). However, optimal conditions for *ex vivo* stimulation and culture of T-lymphocytes, which bear no or low risk of interference with the T-cell physiology, are still to be defined.

Selection marker

A selection step is necessary to ensure exclusive infusion of suicide gene-modified cells. On the other hand, almost 100% retrovirus-mediated gene transfer into primary T-cells could be an alternative [1,18,20]. However, gene transfer rates this high may be impaired by the association of the gene-modified cells with multiple integrations in so significant a proportion that a higher risk of insertional mutagenesis may ensue.

In clinical studies, two different systems for selection of suicide gene-modified T-cells have been exploited so far. TIBERGHIEN and co-workers used the neomycin phosphotransferase gene (neo^R), and 5 days of *in vitro* selection with G418, to obtain pure cell populations [25]. The effectiveness and safety of this system has been assessed in many clinical studies. However, long *in vitro* selection, as required with neo^R, may impair T-cell functions, and, moreover, the neo^R gene product has been reported to be immunogenic in man [26].

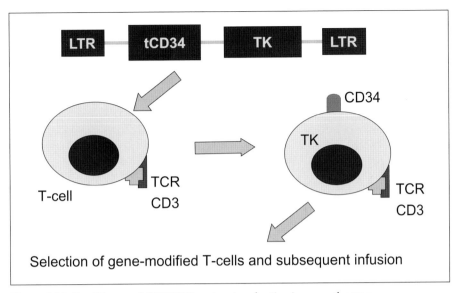

Figure 6.4-2 Possible use of tCD34/TK vectors in adoptive immunotherapy.

BORDIGNON's group developed a truncated version of the low-affinity nerve growth factor receptor (ΔLNGFR) as well as immunoaffinity columns for enrichment of transduced cells [4]. ΔLNGFR allows rapid selection of transduced cells [8,10], using for instance, magnetic cell sorting (MACS), but there is currently no clinical system available for this purpose. Unfortunately, expression of ΔLNGFR has been found on non-transduced cells (referred to as pseudotransduction) [6], thus limiting the possibility of exclusively infusing gene-modified cells. In addition, little is known about possible influences of ΔLNGFR expression on haematopoiesis. Recent publications, and our own data, could not exclude a negative impact of ΔLNGFR-expression, at least in stem and progenitor cells [22, LI et al., submitted]. In summary, both systems have their advantages and disadvantages. Alternative selection markers have yet to be developed.

Recently, we presented a new gene transfer marker, truncated CD34 (tCD34), with a high potential for clinical use [11]. Presently we are constructing several vectors utilizing various co-expression strategies (see above), to ensure efficient expression of both transgenes, i.e. tCD34 and the suicide gene Herpes simplex virus thymidine kinase (HSV-tk) (Fig. 6.4-2). To improve the suicide mechanism, we use an optimized version of HSV-tk [13, CHALMERS et al., submitted] kindly provided by P. TIBERGHIEN.

Adoptive immunotherapy with T-cells has become a powerful approach in the treatment of malignant and viral disease. Introduction of a suicide gene into T-cells is a promising strategy for controlling GvHD, still a potential complication. We conceived a new clinical protocol, in which infusion of suicide gene-modified T-cells is scheduled on day 0 (together with CD34+ cells) and day 60, thereby exploiting the potential of this approach to facilitate engraftment, sustain immune-reconstitution and support an anti-leukaemic effect.

Also, we optimized various technical prerequisites for the clinical application of gene-therapeutic strategies, based on T-lymphocyte utilization. Upcoming clinical trials will provide further understanding as to the feasibility of suicide gene therapy for GvHD.

Acknowledgements

This work was supported by grants to BF (BMBF 0312173 via CellTec), to CB (BMBF 01KV9811) and to ZL (personal DAAD grant).

References

1. Ayuk, F.A., *et al.*: Establishment of an optimised gene transfer protocol for human primary T-lymphocytes according to clinical requirements. Gene Ther 6 (1999) 1788.
2. Barrett, A.J., V. Malkovska: Graft-versus-leukaemia: understanding and using the allo-immune response to treat haematological malignancies. Br J Haematol 93 (1996) 754.
3. Baum, C., et al.: Retroviral vector-mediated gene expression in haematopoietic cells. Curr Opin Mol Ther 1 (1999) 605.
4. Bonini, C., *et al.*: HSV-TK gene transfer into donor lymphocytes for control of allogeneic Graft-versus leukemia. Science 276 (1997) 1719.
5. Champlin, R., *et al.*: Phase I/II study of thymidine kinase (TK)-transduced donor lymphocyte infusion (DLI) in patients with haematologic malignancies. Blood 96 (2000) Suppl.1: abstract 1448.
6. Comoli, P., *et al.*: Measuring gene-transfer efficiency. Nature Med 2 (1996) 1280.
7. Eckert, H.-G., *et al.*: High-dose multidrug resistance in primary human haematopoietic progenitor cells transduced with optimized retroviral vectors. Blood 88 (1996) 3407.
8. Fehse, B., *et al.*: Efficient depletion of alloreactive donor T-lymphocytes based on expression of two activation-induced antigens (CD25 and CD69). Br J Haematol 109 (2000) 644.
9. Fehse, B., *et al.*: Highly-efficient gene transfer with retroviral vectors into human T-lymphocytes on fibronectin (FN). Br J Haematol 102 (1998) 566.
10. Fehse, B., *et al.*: Selective immunoaffinity-based enrichment of CD34+ cells transduced with retroviral vectors containing an intracytoplasmatically truncated version of the human low-affinity nerve growth factor receptor (ΔLNGFR) gene. Hum Gene Ther 8 (1997) 1815.
11. Fehse, B., *et al.*: CD34 splice variant: an attractive marker for selection of gene-modified cells. Molecular Ther 1, (2000) 448.
12. Ferrand, C., *et al.*: Retrovirus-mediated gene transfer in primary T-lymphocytes: influence of the transduction/selection process and of ex vivo expansion on the T-cell receptor beta chain hypervariable region repertoire. Hum Gene Ther 11 (2000) 1151.
13. Garin, M.I., *et al.*: Molecular mechanism for ganciclovir resistance in human T-lymphocytes transduced with retroviral vectors carrying the herpes simplex virus thymidine kinase gene. Blood 97 (2001) 122.
14. Hildinger, M., *et al.*: Dominant selection of haematopoietic progenitor cells with retroviral MDR1-coexpression vectors. Hum Gene Ther 9 (1998) 33.
15. Hildinger, M., *et al.*: Combining myeloprotection and cell surface marking. Gene Ther 6 (1999) 1222.
16. Klump, H., *et al.*: Retroviral vector-mediated expression of HoxB4 in haematopoietic cells using a novel coexpression strategy. Gene Ther (2001) in press.
17. Kolb, H.J., *et al.*: Donor leukocyte transfusions for treatment of recurrent chronic myelogenous leukemia in marrow transplant patients. Blood 76 (1990) 2462.
18. Movassagh, M., *et al.*: Retrovirus-mediated gene transfer into T-cells: 95% transduction efficiency without further in vitro selection. Hum Gene Ther 11 (2000) 1189.
19. Papadopoulos, E.D., *et al.*: Infusion of donor leukocytes to treat Epstein-Barr virus associated lymphoproliferative disorders after allogeneic bone marrow transplantation. N Engl J Med 330 (1994) 1185.

20. POLLOK, K.E., *et al.*: High-Efficiency Gene Transfer into Normal and Adenosine Deaminase-Deficient T-Lymphocytes Is Mediated by Transduction on Recombinant Fibronectin Fragments. J Virol 72 (1998) 4882.
21. RIDDELL, S., *et al.*: Restoration of viral immunity in immunodeficient humans by the adoptive transfer of T-cell clones. Science 257 (1992) 238.
22. ROSENZWEIG, M., *et al.*: Efficient and durable gene marking of haematopoietic progenitor cells in nonhuman primates after nonablative conditioning. Blood 94 (1999) 2271.
23. SLAVIN, S., *et al.*: Immunotherapy of minimal residual disease by immunocompetent T-lymphocytes and their activation by cytokines. Cancer Invest. 10 (1992) 221.
24. TIBERGHIEN, P., *et al.*: Ganciclovir treatment of herpes simplex-thymidine kinase-transduced primary T-lymphocytes: An approach for specific in vivo donor T-cell depletion after bone marrow transplantation? Blood 84 (1994) 1333.
25. TIBERGHIEN, P., *et al.*: Administration of herpes simplex-thymidine kinase-expressing donor T-cells with a T-cell-depleted allogeneic marrow graft. Blood 97 (2001) 63.
26. VERZELETTI, S., *et al.*: Herpes simplex virus thymidine kinase gene transfer for controlled graft-versus-host disease and graft-versus-leukemia: clinical follow-up and improved new vectors. Hum Gene Ther 9 (1998) 2243.

6.5 Genetic Modification of T-Cell Transplants in Compliance with Current GMP

Eckert[1], H. G., B. Fehse[2], C. Lindemann[1], F. Ayuk[2], A. R. Zander[2], A. A. Fauser[1,3], K. Kühlcke[1]

[1] European Institute for Research and Development of Transplantation Strategies (EUFETS), Idar-Oberstein, [2] Bone Marrow Transplantation, Eppendorf University Hospital, Hamburg, [3] Clinic for Bone Marrow Transplantation and Haematology/Oncology, Idar-Oberstein, Germany

Summary

The efficient genetic modification of T-lymphocytes is an essential prerequisite for several gene therapeutic strategies. One attractive approach is the transfer of a suicide gene to control the manipulated cells in case of *graft-versus-host disease* (GvHD) in patients undergoing allogeneic bone marrow transplantation. At present, retroviral vectors are most frequently used in this setting. Recently, we were able to demonstrate that retroviral gene transfer can be substantially improved by preloading viral vectors to tissue culture devices using a low-speed centrifugation step. We here summarize our experience in exploiting this methodology for the generation of gene modified T-cell transplants using a low titre ($\sim 10^5$ IU/ml) clinical grade retroviral vector supernatant.

Introduction

A variety of applications in gene therapy rely on the genetic modification of T-lymphocytes (see articles by THEOBALD, FEHSE, and ABKEN, pp. 175, 181, 187). Current therapeutic protocols are, for example, directed towards genetic and infectious diseases (e.g. ADA-SCID, HIV-infection) or targeting the control of graft-versus-host disease (GvHD) in allogeneic bone marrow transplantation. The latter approaches were introduced by BORDIGNON et al. [2] and TIBERGHIEN et al. [10]. The present status of this kind of therapies is summarized in the article by FEHSE et al., p. 196.

One crucial step for the clinical use of genetically modified T-cells is the engineering of the transplant. To date, conventional retroviral vectors mediating stable integration of the transgene into the genome of the target cell are the vectors of choice for this methodology. Large efforts have been made to optimize retroviral gene transfer into primary T-lymphocytes and substantial progress has been reported in several studies. Especially co-localization strategies with fibronectin or fibronectin fragments and low-speed centrifugation have led to a major improvement in transduction efficiencies reached in small-scale [4,6,8] and large-scale [1] gene transfer experiments. Coating of retroviral vectors to positively charged surfaces of cell culture devices has also been shown [7]. More recently, we were able to demonstrate that it is possible to enrich retroviral vectors on plastic surfaces simply by low speed centrifugation of viral supernatant (KÜHLCKE et al., submitted). This allows us to perform a two-step protocol for the processing of the target cells. First, vectors are pre-loaded by low speed centrifugation to the surface of the respective culture device. Second, target cells are incubated on this pre-loaded surfaces. Processing cells that way exhibits several advantages. Exclusion of the centrifugation step of the target cells is a major improvement in product safety. In addition, the procedure allows control of the ratio of vector particles to target cells (or the resulting MOI). The supernatant of the producer cell line containing metabolites and potentially additional unknown products can be discarded. In addition, pre-loaded vector particles can be washed before introducing them into the protocol step affecting the target cells. In part the technique can be used to compensate for possible low viral titres of clinical grade vector lots by repeating the pre-loading step with fresh supernatant. Use of clinical grade recombinant fibronectin fragments (CH-296) can be omitted from the process, which for a clinical scale transduction is a valid economic aspect. All these features display profound improvements towards a safe and clinically applicable transduction protocol. Consequently, we introduced this technique as a standard in our T-lymphocyte transduction protocol.

Focussing on regulatory requirements in Germany, the engineering of a transplant is regarded as the production of a patient-specific drug and has to be handled according to the German Drug Law. As defined by this law, the production process has to meet the guidelines of *current Good Manufacturing Practice* (cGMP) confirmed through the respective authorities by granting authorization for production.

In accordance with the establishment of a vector production and transduction service for somatic gene therapy phase I/II studies, our unit was authorized to manufacture retroviral vectors in February 2000 and in January 2001, for the purpose of generating gene-modified T-cell transplants.

We here report the results of our final clinical scale evaluation runs for a clinical trial on "The use of gene-modified donor cells in allogeneic bone marrow transplantation (BMT) and peripheral blood stem cell transplantation (PBSCT)", which is introduced and described in detail by FEHSE et al., p. 196. The aim of this study is the control of severe GvHD in allogeneic BMT by a suicide gene mechanism, enabling negative selection of the transduced cells in the patient. Results from our preclinical validation demonstrate that the generation of large numbers of gene-modified T-lymphocytes is feasible, safe and in full compliance with the guidelines of cGMP.

Results and discussion

The retroviral vector which will be used in the clinical trial is shown in Figure 6.5-1. It is based on sequences from the Moloney murine leukaemia virus (Mo-MLV), and carries the herpes simplex virus thymidine kinase cDNA (HSV-tk) as suicide gene linked via an IRES element to the neomycin resistance gene (neoR) for the *in vitro* selection of transduced cells. A volume of 20 l supernatant containing the retroviral vector Mo3TIN was produced in clinical grade quality from a PG13 derived producer cell clone. The supernatant was finally frozen in 100 ml aliquots displaying approximately 10^5 infectious particles/ml after thawing.

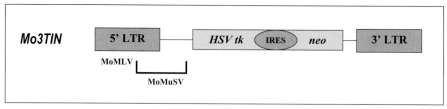

Figure 6.5-1 The retroviral suicide gene vector Mo3TIN.
The retroviral vector Mo3TIN is a Mo-MLV-based vector containing a HSV-tk-IRES-neoR cassette. The herpes simplex virus thymidine kinase cDNA (HSV-tk) is under the control of a Mo-MLV LTR, while the neomycin resistance gene (neoR) is expressed via the internal ribosomal entry site (IRES) of the polio virus. The vector was produced and finally tested as a substance for clinical application at the GMP production facilities at EUFETS, according to a manufacturing authorization given by the German authorities in February 2000.

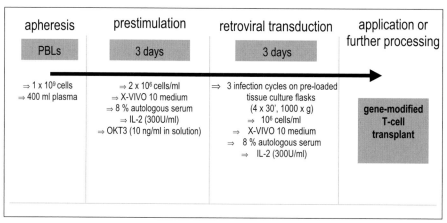

Figure 6.5-2 Protocol for T-lymphocyte transduction on a clinical scale.
Peripheral blood leukocytes were harvested by apheresis from healthy volunteers. A minimum of 1×10^9 cells were harvested, using a minimum of 400 ml plasma. During a three-day pre-stimulation period, cells were incubated at a concentration of 2×10^6/ml in X-VIVO 10 medium (Bio Whittaker, Walkersville, USA) complemented with 8% autologous serum, 300 U/ml IL-2 (Chiron, Amsterdam, Netherlands) and 10 ng/ml OKT3 (Cilag, Neuss). Transduction was carried out in X-VIVO 10 medium supplemented with 8% autologous serum and 300 U/ml IL-2 by three infection cycles on three consecutive days, using the clinical grade vector supernatant. At day one of transduction, cells were adjusted to 1×10^6/ml, before being transferred to vector-pre-loaded, 250 ml tissue culture flasks (Greiner, Frickenhausen). Pre-loading was done by four centrifugation steps (30 min at 1000 x g), each with 25 ml of supernatant.

To demonstrate the clinical feasibility, efficacy and safety of our gene transfer protocol for T-lymphocytes, three evaluation runs were performed on a clinical scale. The transduction protocol is described in detail in Figure 6.5-2. Peripheral blood leukocytes (PBLs) together with a minimum of 400 ml autologous plasma were harvested by apheresis from healthy volunteers. Because conventional retroviral vectors can only integrate into the genome of actively dividing cells, stimulation of the T-cell population is necessary for efficient gene transfer. A combination of IL-2 and the anti-T-cell-receptor-antibody OKT3 was used over

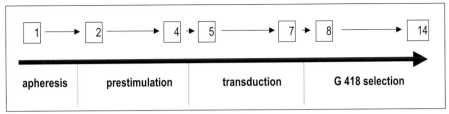

Figure 6.5-3 Cell processing scheme for suicide gene therapy using the vector Mo3TIN. Cells were processed as described in Figure 6.5-1. Clinical lots of vector containing supernatant, filled up to their final volume, were used. After transduction, cells were selected for G418 resistance in X-VIVO 10 medium, supplemented with 8 % human serum and 300 U/ml IL-2 in the presence of 1 mg/ml G418 (Bio Whittaker, Walkersville), for a period of 7 days. During this time, the medium was changed at day 11, while the cells were adjusted to 2 x 10^6/ml. Genomic DNA for real-time quantitative PCR was prepared 48 h after the last transduction.

a three-day period, to force the CD3 positive cells to enter the cell cycle. In addition, 8% autologous serum was added to the culture medium. Earlier studies focussing on the use of different additives clearly favour autologous serum to support *ex vivo* T-cell culture, thus avoiding (in contrast to foetal calf serum) immunological problems at the stage of reinjection of the cells, and for which no additional safety testing is necessary. This pre-stimulation procedure routinely resulted in more than 90% of CD3 positive cells (data not shown). Once growing efficiently, cells tend to form aggregates which should not be disturbed too often during the process by pipetting. Aggregation may facilitate cell to cell interactions via secreted cytokines and is prominent during stimulation and also during the following transduction process.

To compensate for the low viral titre four subsequent low-speed centrifugation pre-loading steps at 1000 x g for 30 min were applied. In addition, cell concentration was adjusted to 10^6/ml at the first day of transduction. IL-2 was kept in the culture medium and renewed every day throughout further cell processing. Three infection cycles were carried out on three consecutive days, by transferring the cell suspension to a new pre-loaded cell culture vessel, once each day. Forty-eight hours after the last infection cycle, the number of vector integrations per genome was measured by real time quantitative PCR performed on a ABI Prism SDS7700 (Applied Biosystems).

Each evaluation run was started with 2 x 10^8 cells in an initial volume of 100 ml which is suitable for handling and for manipulation steps. The cell processing scheme for the transplants is given in Figure 6.5-3. While the absolute cell numbers remain stable during pre-stimulation, cells amplify 4- to 5-fold during the transduction period, an expression of the efficiency of the stimulation process. A range of 0.2 to 0.35 vector copies per genome of the target cells were obtained in separate independent PCR reactions, either for the HSV-tk-gene or for the neoR (Table 6.5-1). Assuming a Gauss distribution for the occurrence of multiple integrations per cell, and taking into consideration that the overall MOI used was below 1, the results obtained imply that roughly 20–35% of the target cells were transduced with the retroviral vector. Possibly, and in the near future, fluorescence *in situ* hybridization, as a promising tool, will provide more

Table 6.5-1 Results summarized from preclinical evaluation.
Three evaluation runs were performed on a clinical scale, in order to demonstrate and confirm the suitability and specifications of the method. Gene transfer efficacy was estimated by detection of vector integration per genome, by real-time quantitative PCR as described [9]. Overall cell numbers resulting from cell processing were determined by trypan blue exclusion.

Scale	Donor	Cell no. (at start)	Cell no. (after G418 selection)	Titre (IU/ml)	Vectors/genome (after transduction)
Clinical	A	2×10^8	1.5×10^9	$\sim 10^5$	0.35
Clinical	B	2×10^8	2.1×10^9	$\sim 10^5$	0.20
Clinical	C	2×10^8	7×10^8	$\sim 10^5$	0.27

explicit data on the single cell level. Using vector supernatants of only 2- to 5-fold higher titres, transduction efficiency of up to one vector copy per genome could be obtained (data not shown).

G418 selection was applied on the transduced cell pool at a concentration of 1 mg/ml G418 (active substance) over a period of seven days, *ex vivo* culture. Proliferation of transduced cells, and cell death of the non-transduced fraction, resulted in a small overall increase in the absolute cell number during this time. Possibly due to the variability in the donor material, we obtained 7 to 21 x 10^9 transduced cells for reinfusion (see table 6.5-1). Interestingly, highest gene transfer efficiency was not correlated to highest T-cell output. Since in the planned clinical trial 5 x 10^6 transduced cells/kg body weight will constitute a transplant, the resulting cell number ought to be large enough to freeze two to three T-cell transplants, thus allowing for a donor lymphocyte infusion in case of relapse.

Examining the cell pool for HSV-tk function after the selection process, we observed that the vast majority of the cells were sensitive to ganciclovir (data not shown). Cell killing of less than 100% can sufficiently be explained by the appearance of a non-functional splice variant of the thymidine kinase [5].

In summary, we were able to show that the transduction protocol we developed for transduction of T-lymphocytes on a clinical scale is suitable for generating large numbers of gene modified cells. In order to preserve the T-cell repertoire, the most important feature is an initially high gene transfer efficacy, itself strongly related to an optimized pre-loading procedure, warranting, subsequently, the co-localization of vector particles and target cells.

For future clinical trials, vector design and positive selection strategies have to be improved in order to shorten the time of *ex vivo* cell culture, because of its main influence on T-cell function.

References

1. AYUK, F.A., *et al.*: Establishment of an optimised gene transfer protocol for human primary T-lymphocytes according to clinical requirements. Gene Ther 6 (1999) 1788–1792.
2. BONINI, C., *et al.*: HSV-TK gene transfer into donor lymphocytes for control of allogeneic graft-versus-leukemia. Science 276 (1997) 1719–1724.

3. BUNNELL, B.A., *et al.*: High-efficiency retroviral-mediated gene transfer into human and nonhuman primate peripheral blood lymphocytes. Proc Natl Acad Sci USA 92 (1995) 7739–7743.

4. FEHSE, B., *et al.*: Selective immunoaffinity-based enrichment of CD34$^+$ cells transduced with retroviral vectors containing an intracytoplasmatically truncated version of the human low-affinity nerve growth factor receptor (deltaLNGFR) gene. Hum Gene Ther 10 (1997) 1815–1824.

5. GARIN M.I., *et al.*: Molecular mechanism for ganciclovir resistance in human T-lymphocytes transduced with retroviral vectors carrying the herpes simplex virus thymidine kinase gene. Blood 97 (2001) 122–129.

6. HANENBERG, H., *et al.*: Colocalization of retrovirus and target cells on specific fibronectin fragments increases genetic transduction of mammalian cells. Nature Med 2 (1996) 876–882.

7. HENNEMANN, B., *et al.*: High-efficiency retroviral transduction of mammalian cells on positively charged surfaces. Hum Gene Ther 11 (2000) 43–51.

8. POLLOK, K.E., *et al.*: High-efficiency gene transfer into normal and adenosine deaminase-deficient T-lymphocytes is mediated by transduction on recombinant fibronectin fragments. J Virol 72 (1998) 4882–4892.

9. SCHIEDLMEIER, B., *et al.*: Quantitative assessment of retroviral gene transfer of the human multidrug resistance-1 gene to human mobilized peripheral blood progenitor cells engrafting in NOD/SCID mice. Blood 95 (2000) 1237–1248.

10. TIBERGHIEN, P., *et al.*: Administration of herpes simplex-thymidine kinase-expressing donor T cells with a T-cell-depleted allogeneic marrow graft. Blood 97 (2001) 63–72.

6.6 Adoptive Immunotherapy in Chimeras

Kolb*, H. J., C. Schmid, M. Schleuning, O. Stoetzer, X. Chen,
A. Woiciechowski, M. Roskrow, M. Weber, W. Guenther, G. Ledderose

Clinical Cooperative Group Haematopoietic Cell Transplantation, Dept. of Medicine III,
Klinikum University of Munich-Großhadern, and GSF-National Research Center for
Environment and Health, Munich, Germany

* To whom correspondence should be addressed (Kolb@med3.med.uni-muenchen.de)

Summary

The use of donor lymphocytes for the treatment of recurrent leukaemia has changed the prospects of haematopoietic stem cell transplantation [2]. Anti-leukaemic principles of myeloablative conditioning have been replaced by adoptive immunotherapy. Experiments in dogs showed that graft-versus-host tolerance can be induced by depletion of T-cells from the graft, and donor lymphocytes could be transfused without graft-versus-host disease (GvHD) later than 60 days after transplantation [12]. In dogs, donor lymphocytes converted mixed chimerism into complete chimerism, transferred immunity to tetanus from the donor to the host, and improved the response to diphtheria toxoid. Donor lymphocytes eliminated leukaemia in patients with recurrent chronic myelogenous leukaemia (CML) after allogeneic bone marrow transplantation [14]. The analysis of the results of centres of the European Cooperative Group of Blood and Marrow Transplantation (EBMT) revealed best results in cytogenetic and haematologic relapses of CML, intermediate results in transformed phase CML, acute myeloid leukaemia (AML) and myelodysplastic syndromes (MDS), and poor results in acute lymphoblastic leukaemia (ALL) [16]. Complications of the treatment were GvHD and myelosuppression. Both absence of chimerism [25] and presence of GvHD were adverse factors for a response. In CML, the graft-versus-leukaemia effect (GvL) correlated with the severity of GvHD, but responses were also seen in patients without GvHD. However, GvL was limited to patients with an allogeneic donor, and failed in patients with a monozygotic twin donor. Antigen presentation was improved by treatment with cytokines. In particular, the combination of interferon-α (IFN-α) and GM-CSF improved the expression of both HLA class I and II antigens and of CD 40 and CD 80 [5]. Preliminary results confirm the beneficial effect of GM-CSF and IFN-α in patients with recurrent CML refractory to donor lymphocytes.

The possibility of differentiation from dendritic cells as professional antigen-presenting cells is common to CML and AML. The leukaemic origin of dendritic cells in culture was shown by FISH analysis, showing the characteristic chromosomal aberration. In AML, the combination of GM-CSF, IL-4, TNF-α and FLT3-L was particularly effective in inducing dendritic cells from AML blasts [33]. The culture was effective in 70 per cent of patients, and included patients with complex karyotypes. In patients with recurrent AML after allogeneic transplantation, the success of donor lymphocyte transfusions is limited because of poor antigen presentation of the blasts and rapid progression of the disease.

We have used low-dose cytosine arabinoside as mild chemotherapy for halting progression of the disease. Mobilized blood was transfused as a preparation of stem cell enriched donor lymphocytes, and GM-CSF was applied for 14–28 days after transfusion. As a result, antigen presentation was optimized by induction of dendritic cells from AML blasts and substitution of dendritic cells from the graft. The response rate was improved from 25 to 67 per cent and the actuarial probability of survival is 25 per cent at 4 years [26]. However, GvHD as well as extramedullary relapses remain as therapeutic problems. An improvement of the results is expected from the immunization of donor cells against minor histocompatibility antigens, expressed on haematopoietic progenitor cells. Sensitized donor lymphocytes should be transduced with a suicide gene, killing the cells in case of severe GvHD. Experiments in dogs are in progress.

Logistic problems limit the use of second donations from unrelated donors and favour family donors. Therefore, regimens for transplantation from HLA-haploidentical family members are being developed. The combination of marrow on day 0 and CD6-depleted mobilized blood on day 6 has shown promising results on otherwise refractory leukaemia [13]. CD6-negative marrow as well as mobilized blood preparations contain a population of natural suppressor cells that suppress mixed lymphocyte reactions and cytotoxic T-cell reactions. However, recurrent immune deficiency and recurrent infections still remain as a problem yet to be solved.

The treatment of leukaemia and neoplastic diseases has changed during the last decades. Bone marrow transplantation, once thought an experimental procedure in selected cases of extremely poor prognosis, has become standard treatment for a variety of diseases [10,23]. The progress of haematopoietic transplantation is related to several areas of improvement: the availability of a donor, the expansion of the source of stem cells, the better diagnosis and treatment of infections, as well as the use of adoptive immunotherapy and less intensive conditioning regimens. Ten years ago, the procedure was limited to a minority of patients with an HLA-identical sibling; today, more than 80 per cent of patients find a suitable donor in internationally available donor registries. The use of mobilized blood as the source of stem cells [27] has improved the number of suitable donors and the amount of available CD34-positive cells as putative stem cells. Early diagnosis of cytomegalovirus (CMV) infections and pre-emptive treatment has decreased the severe complications of CMV disease. The use of donor lymphocytes for the treatment of recurrent or residual leukaemia has stimulated the search for less intensive conditioning regimens [8,18], securing transplantation in patients who would not have been eligible in the past. The dilemma between induction of transplantation tolerance by depletion of T-cells and the beneficial effect of T-cells on residual leukaemia has prompted us to investigate, in dogs, whether the procedure can be separated into two steps: (i) transplantation of T-cell depleted marrow and (ii) transfusion of donor lymphocytes (DLT) for restitution of immunity.

Experiments in dogs

Depletion of T-cells from the marrow by treatment with absorbed antithymo-cyte globulin (ATG) prevents GvHD in DLA-identical littermates, and transfusion of donor lymphocytes on days 1 and 2 as well as days 21 and 22 induces fatal GvHD. However, transfusion on days 61 and 62 does not produce GvHD, and the animals survive. Prior to transfusion, these animals were mixed lymphoid and myeloid chimeras, and became complete chimeras thereafter [12]. The donors were immunized against tetanus toxoid, and, after DLT, the recipients developed antibody titres which persisted for more than 3 years after booster injections. Transfused and non-transfused animals were immunized against diphtheria toxoid as a new antigen. Transfused dogs developed significantly higher antibody titres than animals which had not been transfused.

These experiments indicate that, two months after transplantation, tolerance allowing DLT without the risk of GvHD is established. Moreover, residual haematopoietic cells of the host are eliminated without GvHD. Similar results were obtained in a leukaemia model in mice [11].

Results of donor lymphocyte transfusions in CML

Three patients with recurrent CML after allogeneic marrow transplantation were treated with DLT in 1988 and 1989 [15]. They are still in haematologic and molecular remission of CML. The results were confirmed by others [3,7,9,17,21, 22,28], and the analysis of the results of centres of the European Cooperative Group of Blood and Marrow Transplantation (EBMT) showed best results in cytogenetic and haematologic relapses of CML, intermediate results in transformed phase CML, acute myeloid leukaemia (AML) and myelodysplastic syndromes (MDS), and poor results in acute lymphoblastic leukaemia (ALL) [16]. Complications of the treatment were GvHD and myelosuppression. Both absence of chimerism [25] and presence of GvHD were adverse factors for a response. In CML the graft-versus-leukaemia effect (GvL) correlated with the severity of GvHD, but responses were also seen in patients without GvHD. However, GvL was limited to patients with an allogeneic donor, and failed in patients with a monozygotic twin donor. Antigen presentation was improved by treatment with cytokines. In particular, the combination of interferon-α (IFN-α) and GM-CSF improved the expression of both HLA class I and II antigens and of CD 40 and CD 80 [5]. Preliminary results confirm the beneficial effect of GM-CSF and IFN-α in patients with recurrent CML refractory to donor lymphocytes.

Prevention of GvHD was achieved by two methods without ablating the GvL effect: depleting CD8-positive T-cells from the transfusion [1,9], and using escalating doses of DLT [17] starting at a dose of 2×10^6 lymphocytes per kg. The escalating dose schedule has significantly lowered the risk of GvHD. Patients should be surveyed by regular quantitative RT-PCR for bcr/abl, and in case of persisting or recurrent positivity, the proposed schedule should be a starting dose of 2×10^6 lymphocytes per kg from unrelated donors, or 1×10^7 lymphocytes per kg from an HLA-identical sibling donor. Doses are escalated if there is no GvHD within 30 days or no response within 60 days.

Results of donor lymphocyte transfusions in AML

The EBMT results indicated inferior responses in patients with recurrent AML after DLT. Patients in whom chemotherapy had not induced remission showed a response rate of 25 per cent, with very few cases surviving more than 4 years. Only limited data were available on the FAB subtype and cytogenetic analyses in these patients. With these limitations, the FAB subtype did not influence the response, and a proportion of patients with unfavourable karyotypes did respond to this form of treatment.

Poor antigen presentation as well as rapid progression of disease were considered the major obstacles to adoptive immunotherapy in recurrent AML. Improvement of antigen presentation and production of cytotoxic T-cells against autologous blasts were studied *in vitro*. The combination of GM-CSF, IL-4, TNF-α and FLT3-L was particularly effective in inducing dendritic cells from AML blasts [33]. The culture was effective in 77 per cent of patients and included patients with complex karyotypes. Specific cytotoxic T-cells against autologous blasts were produced in more than 60 per cent of these patients.

We used low-dose cytosine arabinoside as mild chemotherapy for halting progression of the disease. Mobilized blood was transfused as a preparation of stem-cell-enriched donor lymphocytes, and GM-CSF was applied for 14–28 days after transfusion. Consequently, antigen presentation was optimized by induction of dendritic cells from AML blasts as well as substitution of dendritic cells derived from CD34-positive cells of the graft. The response rate was improved from 25 to 67 per cent, and the actuarial probability of survival is 25 per cent at 4 years [26]. However, GvHD and extramedullary relapses persist as therapeutic problems. In some patients, low-dose cytosine arabinoside is not effective in halting disease progression, and more intensive chemotherapy, including anthracyclins, is necessary. In these cases, severe GvHD may develop following transfusion of mobilized blood cells and treatment with GM-CSF. Moreover, GM-CSF may mobilize blasts from the marrow into peripheral blood. As a result, GM-CSF has to be stopped, and in case of severe GvHD immuno-suppressive treatment with steroids, cyclosporine A and azathioprine or other drugs has to be started. Unfortunately, leukaemia may recur during immuno-suppressive treatment, leaving few therapeutic options. An improvement is expected from the immunization of donor cells against minor histocompatibility antigens expressed on haematopoietic progenitor cells [19]. They should not react against other tissues of the patient and thus circumvent GvHD. Sensitized donor lymphocytes should be transduced with a suicide gene effective in killing the cells in case of severe GvHD.

Responses to DLT have been reported for several other diseases such as multiple myeloma, chronic lymphatic leukaemia and non-Hodgkin's lymphoma of low-grade malignancy. In these disorders, slow disease progression and response to IFN-α prevail. At present, it is not known whether mature B-lymphocytes, common to all of them, are effective in antigen presentation to allogeneic lymphocytes or whether the relevant antigens are presented by other blood cells or by the graft.

Any conclusions on the treatment of solid tumors with adoptive immuno-therapy are premature, but the possibility exists that neoplasia, as renal cell cancer, breast cancer or ovarian cancer, respond to allogeneic transplants because of an immune graft-versus-tumor effect [6].

Adoptive immunotherapy against viral infections has been successful in the case of Epstein-Barr virus (EBV) [20,24] and cytomegalovirus (CMV) infections [29]. In these cases, very few unmodified T-cells were effective in the treatment of EBV-associated lymphoma in transplant patients, but severe GvHD was a problem. CD8-positive T-cell clones were effective in preventing CMV disease, but the clones did not survive without the help of CD4-positive T-cells. Lines of T-cells, comprising CD8- and CD4-positive cells, survived in the transplanted patients, and were reactivated with reactivation of EBV.

Transplantation from HLA-haploidentical family members

The number of suitable donors has greatly increased in the last decade, because of the existing registries of unrelated donors. However, problems due to logistics limit the use of second donations from unrelated donors. Therefore, regimens for transplantation from family members sharing one HLA-haplotype and differing in 0–3 HLA-antigens (A, B, DR) of the second haplotype are being developed. The combination of bone marrow on day 0 and CD6-depleted mobilized blood on day 6 achieved promising results on otherwise refractory leukaemia [13]. CD6-negative marrow, and mobilized blood preparations contain a population of natural suppressor cells that suppress mixed lymphocyte reactions and cytotoxic T-cell reactions. Suppression was exhibited by the CD8-positive subset of CD6-negative cells, and was abrogated by depletion of CD8-positive cells; not, however, by the depletion of NK-cells or monocytes. However, recurrent immune deficiency and recurrent infections persist as problems to be solved. The 2-year actuarial survival is 22%, the relapse rate 60%. Infections, however, present therapeutic problems. Future attempts will be directed to transplantation at an earlier stage of the disease and better prevention of infections by improving immune reconstitution.

Future prospects of adoptive immunotherapy

Haematopoietic cell transplantation has come a long way from bone marrow transplantation to adoptive immunotherapy in chimeras. However, the mechanisms of adoptive immunotherapy in chimeras are still far from being understood. The immunobiology of leukaemia, other neoplastic diseases and viral infections has to be studied in human patients. Furthermore, the mechanism of immune tolerance, immune reactivity against normal cells, and transfer of immunity can be studied in animal experiments.

Immunization of donor T-cells against minor histocompatibility antigens of the recipient is currently studied in dogs. Compared to naive T-cells, sensitized cells convert mixed chimerism to complete chimerism much faster. Tests have been developed to demonstrate cellular immunity to haematopoietic progenitor cells *in vitro*, allowing the definition of minor antigens in the dog [30]. The incidence of severe GvHD, post transfusion of sensitized donor lymphocytes into stable chimeras may be 30–50 per cent [31]. The percentage is expected to be higher in human patients, since patients and their donors are exposed to a multiplicity of histocompatibility and viral antigens in their lifetime. Preventive measures against severe GvHD are necessary.

Modification of donor lymphocytes with a suicide gene is the most promising way of prevention. T-cells of the donor are infected with a replication-deficient retrovirus carrying the herpes simplex thymidine kinase gene; this gene phosphorylates ganciclovir, and the resulting nucleotide leads to a stop of DNA polymerization during cell division [4]. Current problems of the method are the altered immune reactivity of transduced T-cells, immune reactions against the viral protein, rejection of the transduced cells and, eventually, altered sensitivity of transduced cells to ganciclovir due to splice variants of the gene. We have studied the method in the dog and found a good immune reactivity of transduced canine T-cells *in vitro*. Transfusion of transduced T-cells into a canine chimera resulted in complete chimerism and transfer of immunity to tetanus toxoid, but impeding the detection of transduced cells which could only be achieved by PCR [32].

Adoptive immunotherapy in chimeras is a promising way of treating leukaemia and, possibly, solid tumours. In particular, the immune reactivity against leukaemias and neoplasia otherwise refractory to chemotherapy offers new perspectives in haematology and oncology.

References

1. ALYEA, E.P., *et al.*: Toxicity and efficacy of defined doses of CD4+ donor lymphocytes for treatment of relapse after allogeneic bone marrow transplantation.. Blood 91 (1998) 3671–3677.
2. ANTIN J.H.: Graft-versus-leukemia: no longer an epiphenomenon. Blood 82 (1993) 2273–2277.
3. BAR B.M.A.M., *et al.*: Donor leukocyte infusions for chronic myeloid leukemia relapsed after allogeneic bone marrow transplantation. J Clin Oncol 11 (1993) 513–519.
4. BONINI, C., *et al.*: HSV-TK gene transfer into donor lymphocytes for control of allogeneic graft-versus-leukemia. Science 276 (1997) 1719–1724.
5. CHEN, X., *et al.*: Interferon alpha in combination with GM-CSF induces the differentiation of leukaemic antigen-presenting cells that have the capacity to stimulate a specific anti-leukaemic cytotoxic T-cell response from patients with chronic myeloid leukaemia. Br J Haematol 111(2) (2000) 596–607.
6. CHILDS, R., *et al*: Regression of metastatic renal-cell carcinoma after nonmyeloablative allogeneic peripheral-blood stem-cell transplantation. N Engl J Med 343(11) (2000) 750–758.
7. COLLINS, R.H., *et al.*: Donor leukocyte infusions in 140 patients with relapsed malignancy after allogeneic bone marrow transplantation. J Clin Oncol 15 (1997) 433–444.
8. GIRALT, S., *et al.*: Engraftment of allogeneic haematopoietic progenitor cells with purine analog-containing chemotherapy: harnessing graft-versus-leukemia without myeloablative therapy. Blood 89 (1997) 4531–4536.
9. GIRALT, S., *et al.*: CD8-depleted donor lymphocyte infusion as treatment for relapsed chronic myelogenous leukemia after allogeneic bone marrow transplantation. Blood 86 (1995) 4337–4343.
10. GOLDMAN, J.M., *et al.*: Allogeneic and autologous transplantation for haematological diseases, solid tumours and immune disorders: current practice in Europe in 1998. Bone Marrow Transplant 21 (1998) 1–7.
11. JOHNSON, B.D., *et al.*: Truitt: Delayed infusion of normal donor cells after MHC-matched bone marrow transplantation provides an antileukemia reaction without graft-versus-host disease. Bone Marrow Transplant 11 (1993) 329–336.
12. KOLB, H.J., *et al.*: Adoptive immunotherapy in canine chimeras. Transplantation 63 (1997) 430–436.
13. KOLB, H.J., *et al.*: CD-6 negative blood stem cells facilitating HLA-haploidentical transplantation in the treatment of advanced leukemia. Blood 96[11] (2000) 208a–208a (Abstract).

14. KOLB, H.J., *et al.*: Donor leukocyte transfusions for treatment of recurrent chronic myelogenous leukemia in marrow transplant patients. Blood 76 (1990) 2462–2465.

15. KOLB, H.J., *et al.*: Treatment of recurrent chronic myelogenous leukemia posttransplant with interferone alpha (INF-α) and donor leukocyte transfusions. Blut 61 (1990) 122–122.

16. KOLB, H.J., *et al.*: Graft-versus-leukemia effect of donor lymphocyte transfusions in marrow-grafted patients. Blood 86 (1995) 2041–2050.

17. MACKINNON, S., *et al.*: Adoptive immunotherapy evaluating escalating doses of donor leukocytes for relapse of chronic myeloid leukemia after bone marrow transplantation: separation of graft-versus-leukemia responses from graft-versus-host disease. Blood 86 (1995) 1261–1268.

18. MCSWEENEY, P.A., *et al.*: Haematopoietic cell transplantation in older patients with haematologic malignancies: replacing high-dose cytotoxic therapy with graft-versus-tumor effects. Blood 97(11) (2001) 3390–3400.

19. MUTIS, T., *et al.*: Feasibility of immunotherapy of relapsed leukemia with ex vivo generated cytotoxic T-lymphocytes specific for haematopoietic system-restricted minor histo-compatibility antigens. Blood 93(7) (1999) 2336–2341.

20. PAPADOPOULOS, E.B., *et al.*: Infusions of donor leukocytes to treat Epstein-Bar virus-associated lymphoproliferative disorders after allogeneic bone marrow transplantation. N Engl J Med 330 (1994) 1185–1191.

21. PORTER, D.L., *et al.*: Induction of graft-versus-host disease as immunotherapy for relapsed chronic myeloid leukemia. New Engl J Med 330 (1994) 100–106.

22. VAN RHEE, F., *et al.*: Relapse of chronic myeloid leukemia after allogeneic bone marrow transplant: The case for giving donor leukocyte transfusions before the onset of haematological relapse. Blood 83 (1994) 3377–3383.

23. RIZZO, J.D.: 1998 IBMTR/ABMTR (Statistical Center, Medical College of Wisconsin, Milwaukee, WI, USA). Summary Slides on State-of-the-Art in Blood & Marrow Transplantation. ABMTR Newsletter 5[1] (1998) 4–10.

24. ROONEY, C.M., *et al.*: Control of virus-induced lymphoproliferation: Epstein-Barr virus-induced lymphoproliferation and host immunity. Mol Med Today 1997; 3(1):24–30.

25. SCHATTENBERG, A., *et al.*: In relapsed patients after lymphocyte depleted bone marrow transplantation the percentage of donor T-lymphocytes correlates well with the outcome of donor leukocyte infusion. Leuk Lymphoma 32(3–4) (1999) 317–325.

26. SCHMID, C., *et al.*: Treatment of recurrent acute leukemia after marrow transplantation with donor cells and GM-CSF. Blood 94[10 Suppl. 1] (1999) 668a–668a.

27. SCHMITZ, N., *et al.*: Randomised trial of filgastrim-mobilised peripheral blood progenitor cell transplantation in lymphoma patients. Lancet 347 (1996) 353–357.

28. SLAVIN, S., *et al.*: Allogeneic cell therapy with donor peripheral blood cells and recombinant human interleukin-2 to treat leukemia relapse after allogeneic bone marrow trans-plantation. Blood 8(7) (1996) 2195–2204.

29. WALTER, E.A., *et al.*: Reconstitution of cellular immunity against cytomegalovirus in recipients of allogeneic bone marrow by transfer of T-cell clones from the donor. N Engl J Med 333 (1995) 1038–1044.

30. WEBER, M., *et al.*: CFU-suppression by T-Cells primed with DLA-identical dendritic cells. Bone Marrow Transplant 25(Suppl. 1) (2000) S23-abstract.

31. WEIDEN, P.L., *et al.*: Infusion of donor lymphocytes into stable canine radiation chimeras: Implications for mechanism of transplantation tolerance. J Immunol 116 (1976) 1212–1219.

32. WEISSINGER, E.M., *et al.*: Expression of HSV-TK suicide gene in primary T-lymphocytes: The dog as a preclinical model. Cytokines, Cellular & Molecular Therapy 6(1) (2000) 25–33.

33. WOICIECHOWSKY, A., *et al.*: Leukemic dendritic cells generated in the presence of FLT3 ligand have the capacity to stimulate an autologous leukaemia-specific cytotoxic T-cell response from patients with acute myeloid leukaemia. Leukemia 15 (2001) 246–255.

Index

Page numbers in *italics* refer to figures and/or tables.